I0486763

WRONG WAY BRAIN

Reflections On and About a Left-Brain Society

HELENA MOORE, PH.D.

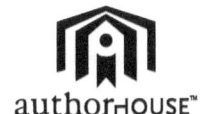

authorHOUSE™

1663 LIBERTY DRIVE, SUITE 200
BLOOMINGTON, INDIANA 47403
(800) 839-8640
WWW.AUTHORHOUSE.COM

First published by AuthorHouse 12/21/05

ISBN: 1-4208-8030-6 (sc)

Printed in the United States of America
Bloomington, Indiana

This book is printed on acid-free paper.

Dedicated to the Spirit
and the Memory of
Helen Petres Brookins

ACKNOWLEDGMENTS

Thank you to everyone who has had a part in bringing about the reality of this little book. Without Amy Eastham in Cazenovia, NY, there is no telling how long it would have taken for me to begin my educational journey: Cazenovia College, which then was Cazenovia Junior College; Antioch College; Syracuse University; Fairfield University; the Psychoanalytic Center; Union Institute, which at the time of my admittance was The Union for Experimenting Colleges and Universities; and on from there. Thank you to all my teachers, including Pieter Kors, who made me aware of what I wanted to do with the rest of my life.

Jean Balderston; Paula Stewart, now Paula Ohanesian; Bradley Coates; Kathy Garlick; Gwen Billups-Newton and Nancy Slater were some of those who gave me important personal support as these essays were being incubated. Longtime friends and colleagues Marianne Berson and Helen McDermott were pillars of support throughout the honing of what became the final manuscript. Thank you.

Assistance from the Ramapo Catskill Library System was invaluable. My appreciation to the librarians at the Ethelbert Crawford Library in Monticello, and to the librarians in the extended system. My thanks especially to Sharon Stanton, who showed me the buttons on the computer which gave what seemed like magical access to the world of books available through the Internet.

I also want to thank Penguin Group (USA) Inc. for permission to use the twin sailors paragraph from Marilyn Ferguson's *The Aquarian Conspiracy*, published by J.P. Tarcher, Inc., which appears in the Introduction.

Last, and most important, indelible admiration and respect go to all who keep their focus on whole brain values in spite of needing to live and work within left brain constraints.

Helena Moore
Forestburgh, NY

CONTENTS

INTRODUCTION
Regarding Our Two Thought Systems

When I began my doctoral studies more than twenty years ago, I wanted to investigate different thinking styles. What is commonly known today about the different ways of processing by the two hemispheres of the Neocortex was then only on the cusp of being known by the layperson. I was recognizing the output of each of the hemispheres without knowing how specific the reason was behind the output. It wasn't long into my search before the two protagonists of my study emerged.

Over the past couple of decades it has become common knowledge that we house two separate ways of thinking inside our skulls, one digital, one analogic, like two separate computers, connected, yet each processing information in its own separate way. While we can give a list of all the adjectives describing each of the computer's skills (left: logical, mathematical, organizational, etc.—right: creative, conceptualizing, synthesizing, etc.) it seems to elude us that we have a choice as to which computer will take precedence in taking care of the affairs of living. More than one philosopher has pointed out that we have taken a wrong turn in evolution, and the way we have learned to use the binary system in our brain is responsible. Susanne Langer and Donald Carr are just two representatives of this cadre, and Bob samples is just one of the people who has pointed out that what has gone wrong in the evolutionary process is the result of the acculturation process.

"The left brain thinks, the right brain <u>knows,</u>" and other such prognostications elicited, dot by dot, enough of a whole picture to explain the reasons why it is so difficult for some of us to understand others among us, as though we are speaking the same words, but in a different language.

While it has become clear that the right hemisphere person is better able to size up a situation, and faster, something that was learned in time put a special kind of spin on this knowledge. It is the right hemisphere that tends to see the whole picture, yet the person who is strongly into using more of the attributes of the left hemisphere tends to take charge, often denigrating the right hemisphere's perspective. With the exception proving the rule, those who are able to see the whole picture are not those who are in charge.

These essays have been written with a combination of humility and hubris—humility because the field of brain research is in its infancy, and some of the current theories are in conflict with one another. Will the brain ever be fully known and understood? But without the hubris, most of these essays would never have been written. The genesis of the hubris is that before I knew why there are different thinking styles, I knew that there are different thinking styles. Much as the application of water to wood makes the grain in the wood more visible, certain things became more clear as more was learned about hemispheric differences. The most cogent description I have found about the differences in how the two hemispheres function is from Marilyn Ferguson's *The Aquarian Conspiracy*:

Our plight might be compared to the long, long journey of twin sailors. One is a verbal, analytical fellow, the other mute and sometimes dreamy. The verbal partner earnestly calculates with the aid of his charts and instruments. His brother, however, has an uncanny ability to predict storms, changing currents, and other navigational conditions, which he communicates by signs, symbols, drawings. The analytical sailor is afraid to trust his brother's advice because he can't imagine its source. Actually, the silent sailor has wireless, instantaneous access to a rich data bank that gives him a satellite perspective on the weather. But he cannot explain this complex system with his limited ability to communicate details. And his talkative, "rational" brother usually ignores him anyway. Frustrated, he often stands by helplessly while their craft sails head-on into disaster. (p. 298)

This is a testament to the strong suggestion that we may be using our brains the wrong way. It is taken for granted that we are a "left-brain society." While the left hemisphere is a marvelous tool, we should not be putting the tool in charge. It is the right hemisphere that we need to put back in charge—evolutionarily it was in charge before we developed the tool of written language. And it appears to be no coincidence that before the left hemisphere began to be in charge that matriarchy preceded what came to be patriarchy.

Split brain research has proved how important it is for the two separate hemispheres to work together. There are marked differences in the way information is processed which affect personality, and thus our collective environment. The right hemisphere is great at knowing what needs to be done, keeping all the elements of a given situation in mind, while the left hemisphere is great at implementation. Value issues, gender issues and political issues are all affected by how we use our collective brain. The right hemisphere wants to cooperate, while the left loves competition. Perhaps the most important thing for us to concentrate on, along with strengthening right hemisphere use, is to increase the facility of the Corpus Callosum, the major connecting commissure between the two halves of the Neocortex, helping the hemispheres to work together. Language need not suffer, nor do all the other tools we have devised with our vast amount of intelligence. It is only a matter of putting our priorities in order.

While we are considering the importance of hemispheric specialization, we should not forget that we will have constant input from our historical brains, which neuroscientist Paul MacLean, M.D. dubbed "the Triune Brain." Like small houses built one on top of another are the Reptilian Brain, which deals with unlearned and preprogrammed behavior including such things as self-preservation and the establishment of territory; the Paleomammalian Brain, made up largely of the Limbic System which has the capacity for emotional expression; and the Neomammalian Brain which boasts the Neocortex. The Neocortex is the particularly human brain which helps to decide how to use all the integral units of our historical heritage. We have it within our cranial equipment to use the whole brain in a more balanced, more creative, more satisfying way. And if we can understand the brain as wonderfully complex, rather than terrifyingly complex, as it has been called, we will have the possibility of a more promising prognosis, for this attitude would have the tendency of putting us, rather than our inventions, in charge. It is up to us how our evolution unfolds.

In many of these essays the names of writers, scientists and philosophers are mentioned so that readers may choose, if desired, to pursue an idea further.

And from time to time in the discussion of hemispheric differences some personal reminiscences are mentioned. Please note in reading these essays that whenever a case history has been mentioned, names and circumstances have been altered to preserve confidentiality.

ANIMALS
Our Antediluvian Roots

Do you ever feel that you identify more with animals than with people? As I drove down a relatively quiet road a few days ago, it was not difficult to identify with the spirit of a tiny kitten who could not have been more than three weeks old. This little creature, out to see the world, came marching toward me down the middle of the road, spiky tail pointing straight up. Another car was coming toward us from down the road. Averting tragedy, I stopped my car, motioned to the oncoming car to slow down, picked up the kitten and put it down near the door of the house to which I had seen what was probably the mother cat running as my car came along.

After getting back in the car and preparing to start it up again, there was that little kitten, right out in the middle of the road again, tiny tail perpendicular to the tiny body, marching down the middle of the road again, as though determined to seek its fortune out there somewhere. This time after picking her up I rang the bell of the house of cats and waited until I could put the little furry thing into the hands of a big burly man. This little cat was destined to have her—or his—way in the world. So be it if this sounds like anthropomorphism, but let us not forget that feelings are from the limbic brain and that animals had the limbic brain before we did.

It seems as though every time I go to the veterinarian's office, having time for a conversation with one or another of the pet owners, that a crusty old man or a timid-looking young woman will state in a firm voice that they like animals better than people. That is not hard to understand. Walt Whitman in his *Leaves of Grass* put it well, about animals: "They do not lie awake in the dark and weep for their sins, They do not make me sick discussing their duty to God, Not one is dissatisfied, not one is demented with the mania of owning things."

It is not unusual for someone who has been despondent and without direction to have been given a spiritual jumpstart by the inimitable spirit of a dog, a cat, or any other representative of the animal kingdom. It is not unusual for a child to have learned about love from a pet—a dog is high on this list. Even a turtle, and even fish in a tank, have been within my repertoire of memories of these humble mental health workers. The owner of a fish tank, let's call her Zelda, had been extremely depressed and lonely because of her inability to make connections with people. Intelligent and beautiful, her lack of self confidence had kept her somewhat isolated, but the artist in her had kept a constant connection with beautiful tropical fish in a medium-sized tank and, intellect riding on the back of feeling, her academic progress had accelerated.

I lost track of Zelda when I relocated. Ten years or so later she phoned me, delighted that she had found me. She wanted me to know how her life had changed. The first thing she told me was that she, who had begun her journey away from depression with a tank of tropical fish, had found herself a dog. Apparently the next logical step in her Unconscious had been a boyfriend. At the point of the phone call she had found time enough in her professional life to marry and have a child.   Somehow, the recognition of the importance of the fish tank so many years ago seems important in that it had been her first conscious connection to life. Her personal evolution had proceeded from there.

Although we have progressed beyond the limbic brain of animals in many ways, including the gifts of speech and the ability to plan, we sacrificed much of the intuitive abilities that animals still retain. We are still young enough in our evolution to recapture some of the intuitive wisdom which we have sacrificed in favor of left brain characteristics, but we need to understand the deficits of the sacrifice. The sometimes uncanny ability of animals to know what is going on even when we don't know is an important part of what makes the connection to them so healing. Not only are they direct and accepting, they are also extremely good listeners, which usually makes them more helpful than people, who sometimes can only give advice.

One of my most influential teachers was InKee, a cat who lived with no sight for half his life of twelve years. He taught me the concepts of endurance, of patience and of courage.   How strange that often it is animals who give us a clear concept of what it can mean to be human.

Countless individuals who have been part of the growing number of the "mentally ill" have begun their road to recovery with animals. Every time I ask myself why that is, whether it is a turtle, a tank of fish, a cat or a dog, I keep coming back to the word "integrity." Carl Rogers long ago pointed out that the more we can honestly be who we are, "the other" is enabled to be him or herself. This maxim applies to more than other people. The integrity of the animals rubs off on us. The emotional reservoir is much deeper than what can be conveyed by words.

Helena Moore, Ph.D.

It is a continuing mystery as to how and why psychotherapy is effective. Sometimes a look can be the key to opening up the door to the psyche, to let mending begin, no matter how many words had come before. It is no coincidence that sometimes those looks are from the animals who love us.

A New Paradigm
The Wisdom of the Right Hemisphere

With roughly 95% of the population the left brain will be the logical, analytical brain; the right brain will be the artistic, holistic hemisphere. All this is metaphorical, because each brain is organized somewhat differently from all other brains. It is the attributes that have been seen as being the province of each hemisphere that are important, rather than strictly right or left. Without the Corpus Callosum, the band of fibers that connects the hemispheres, we would not be able to take advantage of the combined skills of both hemispheres. We need the whole brain, but it is the relative importance of the two hemispheres that is significant.

Because it has language skills, the left hemisphere came to be thought of as the thinking brain, while right brain thinkers have been considered less intelligent than those with more of the left brain skills. Now it is beginning to be recognized by some that right brain skills have an important place in our very survival. We need the wisdom of the right brain skills. While the left brain is verbal, rational, analytical and goal-oriented, the right hemisphere is intuitive, holistic, concrete and spatial. The subtleties of observation which might elude left-brain thinkers are picked up by the right hemisphere thinkers, but because they tend to be non-verbal, their observations, which could be so helpful, often remain unarticulated. Right brain thinkers will see the whole picture—for instance, they will see the forest and the interrelationships of the trees, while the left brain thinkers will only see the individual trees. The late Dr. Roger Sperry, one of the most important brain researchers because of his split brain studies, was one of the first to establish the importance of recognizing the bi-modal brain. According to Dr. Sperry, two modes of thinking, verbal and nonverbal, are represented separately in left and right hemispheres, respectively. He points out that our educational system, as well as science in general, tends to neglect the nonverbal form of intellect. He goes on to say that modern society discriminates against the right hemisphere. In other words, our left-brain society tends to ignore the wisdom of the right hemisphere.

In *The Right Brain* Robert Ornstein comments that modern education tends to be reductionist. He makes a case for the necessity of putting the larger picture in front of the student. While the left hemisphere dictates our social, educational, and political lives, the right brain tends to be silent, and must figure out a way to get across its particular strengths. Presenting more of an overall view to students would encourage the development of right brain interests, and it follows that the result would mean more whole-brain thinking.

It is troubling that brain research has discovered that the left brain, if it does not know an answer, will choose to make something up rather than to say, "I don't know." Furthermore, the left brain tends to put down the attempts of the right brain to give information to the left brain. At times left sees right as insignificant and bothersome. More and more scientists are acknowledging the importance of right brain thinking. In *Fabric of the Mind*, Neurosurgeon Richard Bergland, M.D., refers to the right brain as the seat of the sense of beauty, and perhaps the center of the human mind's highest abilities intellectually. Richard Gerber, M.D., in *Vibrational Medicine*, refers to the right brain as "the Higher Self," and sees dreams as an attempt to integrate the Higher Self and the physical personality.

The essays in this book, one way or another, are all about the importance of being able to change the focus of our attitudes, determined by which brain hemisphere we encourage to take charge. How we evolve as a species (or not) will be determined by how we choose to use our brains. We are still phylogenetically young enough to recapture some of the instinctive wisdom of the right brain which we have neglected in favor of being able to communicate with words. We will not lose our verbal abilities—it is only necessary that we recognize how we are overlooking some important gifts which the metaphorical right hemisphere can contribute. The way we have become accustomed to using the binary system in our brain is responsible for what has been called "a wrong turn in evolution."

It might be a good idea to think in terms of trying to encourage the Corpus Callosum to evolve into a more important part of the Neocortex, presiding over both left and right hemispheres, an executive department to make better use of the varying skills of the left and the right hemispheres. Women, who usually have a larger, more active Corpus Callosum than men, have the advantage of more rapid switching back and forth from analog to digital type of thinking, and thus are more naturally "whole-brain thinkers."

LIFE ON PLANET EARTH
Gaia Weeps

Physicist Mitchell Feigenbaum, while studying the borderline between organized behavior and the chaotic behavior of matter, found that Nature favors just a few patterns. This has been an important insight. Feigenbaum used the computer intensively to explore problems but depended on his intuition for key breakthroughs. Whole brain thinking doesn't get much better than this.

Seeing patterns and identifying important links such as Feigenbaum's are mental endeavors that are best done by individuals. Often, however, breakthroughs such as these have difficulty breaking through the barriers of institutional thinking. Many insightful thinkers have run into rejection and downright derision because of independent thinking. Seeing and understanding what has been outside an already accepted set of understandings has not been popular. In order to follow their individual hypotheses scientists who have been able to step outside the political boundaries of the sciences have often received censure from the scientific community. Even though Thomas Kuhn's *The Structure of Scientific Revolutions* established the importance of being able to understand significantly different ways of thinking, independent thinkers often have had to disengage themselves from the restrictive scientific community in order to follow their own insights.

Just one of these thinkers is David Lovelock. Lovelock is responsible for recognizing that our Earth may be the equivalent of a large pattern of life, though this is difficult for the layperson to see because of the size of the earth and the subtlety of the concept. Just as each of us is more than the sum of our brain, our other organs, our blood and our bones, Earth, called Gaia by the Greeks more than two thousand years ago, might be seen as more than the sum of its parts, such as water, air, rock, and soil, with Gaia's biosphere being the equivalent of our aura. Just as we strive to maintain a regulated body temperature, Gaia has thus far been able to maintain homeostasis, an analogic attempt at keeping a balanced environment. However, much of scientific thought is still based on the assumption that Nature is a lifeless mechanistic system.

Lovelock has recognized Earth as a living unit sustained by interacting with its environment in a vast cooperative endeavor. Lovelock's first book, *Gaia, A New Look at Life on Earth,* offended some scientists because he gave interpretations which were felt to be too personal. For example, at one point he commented that "Gaia likes it cold," meaning that the Earth system seems to operate better at a low temperature. Scientists thought that did not sound scientific. And so, once again, our inventions (in this case scientific methodology) try to take charge of our individual minds. Society seeks conformity, while Nature seeks individuation. Lovelock pointed out that to dare to individuate is to risk being seen as eccentric. In order to gain the attention of scientists, Lovelock in his second book, *The Ages of Gaia,* left out any comments which might have been seen as "philosophical." Lovelock saw that science lacked a wholeness of vision.

For example, he pointed out that there are at least thirty different kinds of biologists, almost proud that they know nothing about the other branches. And that the different kinds of biologists don't talk to each other, while every year new branches develop. He further pointed out that the fragmentation has grown at a time when synthesis is needed more than ever. His story alone urges the private individual to reach beyond the confines of organizational and political propriety.

The ideas of some of our best visionaries become stalemated by the dictates of the policies of the companies for whom they work and by the thinking of society at large. Just one part of the problems confronting Gaia is overpopulation. Some pundits believe that the monogamy of same sex relationships is an attempt by Gaia to reduce the burgeoning birth rate.

Lovelock pointed out that Earth is at risk. While politicians are depending on the self-repairing abilities of Gaia to handle the damage, life cannot repair itself when it is dead. And there is no doubt that Gaia is at risk. One of Lovelock's inventions is the electron capture detector, which gave Rachel Carson the proof she needed concerning the poisoning of the environment, detailed in her 1962 book *Silent Spring*. The electron capture detector provided data proving that pesticide residues were present in every creature of the Earth—*in every creature of the Earth.*

People such as David Lovelock do not have to be as lonely in their thinking today as when his first Gaia book came out in 1979. Even though there is still denial in high places, it is beginning to be more common knowledge that the planet is in big trouble. That global warming is happening has been given visible proof from NASA satellite photographs. In 1979 year-round sea ice which began halfway down the east coast of Greenland, extended over the North Pole and stretched to Siberia has now shrunk by two hundred and fifty million acres.

An EPA report on the state of the environment included a section on climate, in which the President at the time deleted references to a study showing steep increases in global temperatures over the past ten years. Also, more than fifty investigations into Clean Air Act violations had been cancelled. This in spite of a statement in the World Scientists' Call for Action at the Kyoto Climate Summit maintaining that political leadership must introduce incentives that will reward sound practices. Some of our politicians choose to ignore this advice.

One wonders whether power plant operators who are in violation of the Clean Air Act would understand the point of the Anita Kunz cartoon on the cover of *The New Yorker* magazine of October 13, '03 depicting a violating president riding a wild-eyed, terrified-looking steed. A bemused glance at the cartoon strongly suggests that in this case it is the frightened horse that is seeing the whole picture, for the blinders are on the rider, rather than on the horse. A comment attributed to Yogi Berra comes to mind: "We are lost, but we are making good time."

DICHOTOMANIA
Two Eyes, Two Minds

As someone who mentally translated into French all heard conversation when first studying French, and as someone who tended to mentally type all heard conversation into paperless, invisible transcriptions when first learning to type, it came as no surprise that when news of the different tasks of the two neocortical hemispheres became part of a mental armamentarium that it should become habit to separate all thinking into left and right brain thinking. In other words, dichotomania set in.

Dichotomania is the strong tendency to see everything as being the product of either left-brain or right-brain thinking. The triune brain—the reptilian, limbic brain, and neo-cortex—is our heritage. In fact, it is possible that a fixation with the characteristics of the bi-modal brain may be tapping into the antediluvian fixed stare which may well be a relic of the reptilian brain. Use of the whole brain, of course, is normal, but the neo-cortex is what makes us human. And separated into two distinct units as it is, we all tend to favor one hemisphere over the other. While both hemispheres deal with the same things, they deal with these same things in different styles. They process information in distinctly different ways. This difference has been described as digital vs. analogic, or as disciplined and customized vs. spontaneous and intuitively knowing. "The left brain thinks, the right brain knows."

Although approximately ninety-five percent of the population has the language center in the left hemisphere, every brain is organized somewhat differently, so it must be understood that when left-brain thinking and right-brain thinking are being discussed that it is a metaphorical type of discussion. Speaking of types of thinking, lawyers need to be able to use left-brain thinking, and artists need to be right-brain specialists. Both hemispheres are needed, but the important consideration is which hemisphere is the leader. Brain researchers in the 1800's found that injury to the left hemisphere resulted in a loss of language facility. Finding no corresponding aphasia as a result of right hemisphere damage, it was deduced that the left hemisphere was the "thinking brain," because it is the talking brain. This corroborated the already socially approved and politically correct way of interacting with the world, depending on logical states of mind rather than on the recognition of feeling states of mind, as though it were depending on the brain rather than "the heart." Because of the research that has developed from about 1960, there has been a new appreciation for the skull's silent partner, but our social organization still does not know how to let this silent partner earn its right to be respected for its own attributes. Like the poor relation, its input is not encouraged. Native Americans are able to articulate the metaphorical difference. They say, "The white man thinks with his head, while we think from the heart."

If we run down a list of the attributes which have been assigned to the two hemispheres by brain researchers it becomes evident that we may be depriving ourselves of the unrecognized strength of the viewpoint of this silent partner.

The right brain wants to cooperate, the personality of the left will compete. The most important single attribute of right-brain thinking is that it tends to see the whole picture, while the left hemisphere tends to see things analytically and reductively. In psychology, the two modes are represented by gestalt and behaviorism. The right brain, able to see the whole picture, should be the brain to choose when to give free rein to its left counterpart and when to quietly insist on a cooperative stance. In other words, the right hemisphere should be in charge and be able to take advantage of left brain skills, as the left is very good at implementation.

For most of the population, all of the above quietly falls into place. The different brain characteristics do not stand out so distinctly. For a dichotomaniac, however, the challenge is ever present, like finding the hidden Ninas in an Al Hirschfeld cartoon, to find the evidence of the specific characteristics of the two thinking style variables. It becomes apparent that there are great subtleties at work, and that at times it is like a throw of the dice as to which hemisphere's perceptions will be in charge. Once you are on to the stylistic differences, it is not difficult to become a dichotomania junkie.

You will begin to notice that the left hemisphere keeps taking things apart, to deal with things separately, for the left brain is reductionistic, while the right hemisphere keeps trying to deal with all the parts together, for the right brain is holistic. All one need do is to read the newspaper to begin to see the different hemispheres at work, in politics, in education, in religion. While the right brain is considered to be the keeper of a sense of integrity, studies of split brain patients have proved that when the left brain does not know the answer to a problem that it will make something up—integrity is not an issue.

William Wordsworth certainly was in touch with right-brain thinking, although he would not have known what to

---

Helena Moore, Ph.D.

call it: From his poem *The World:* "The world is too much with us; late and soon, Getting and spending, we lay waste our powers: Little we see in Nature that is ours; We have given our hearts away, a sordid boon!"

As for a classical example of left brain input, aided and abetted by right brain creativity, swirling over the heads of some of our formerly most powerful CEO's are the results of too much thinking "from the head." While CEO's are known for their ability to be "whole-brained," the ability of many of the CEO's of large corporations to manipulate their environment marks them as being able to override the whole-picture value system of their metaphorical right hemispheres. Their right could have seen the possible outcome of the manipulations, and billions of dollars of the taxpayers' money would not have been sacrificed.

Need there be a more cogent example of why there needs to be more respect for the kind of thinking that the metaphorical right brain does? Perhaps something positive can come from what has been called dichotomania, perhaps the promotion of a new paradigm of the hemispheres, in that there would be more awareness of the subtle strength of the quiet right hemisphere. The more that we understand the differences in our ability to literally be of two minds about something, the more we will be able to understand the implications of our thinking choices, and of our ability to choose the appropriate thinking style.

We might use our dichotomaniacal thinking to make clear how the switch in leadership of the thinking of the hemispheres might work. An analogy might be to use the world of music: Consider right brain thinking as being a descant to the main melody of left brain themes, then think in terms of the two contrapuntal melodies changing their roles, with the descant becoming the main melody, and left-brain thinking becoming a lovely affirmative descant. True, this would be difficult for left-brain thinkers to do,

16

for the left-brain thinks of itself as the main melody, but once this kind of thinker got the hang of it, the benefits, though subtle, would speak for themselves. Among the subtle benefits would be broader understandings, a difficult thing to categorize, and the ability to be happier, a strange concept in our troubled world.

CHANGE

Leading with the Right Hemisphere

Because spirit is so hard to define, modern medicine has not yet been able to consistently take spirit into consideration in problems of physical or emotional illness. "Spiritual" many times is confused with "religious," and although spiritual is an important part of religious, religious is not necessarily a part of the spiritual. Spirit is in every breath we take, and in every endeavor that we explore. Physical personality has been codified as a manifestation of the soul in chemical clothing.

People often notice that within a day or two of what has been a jolt to them emotionally that they come down with the flu or a bad cold. Lucy, a friend who had been critically injured in a car accident, had been able to have a full recovery, able to walk, run, ski, etc., following a long series of physical therapy treatments. On occasion, however, her knee and ankle would "go out," and the pain would be considerable enough for her to use a cane. Then she began to notice that every time she started limping from the unexpected and unusual pain, the limp would start right after she had endured a blow to her self esteem, thus to her spirit. Every time, when she realized what the "blow" had been, the pain disappeared, as though magically. This is an example of a very fast-acting change in how the etheric body affects the physical body.

In *Vibrational Medicine,* Richard Gerber, M.D. points out that research suggests that changes in the etheric body precede manifestations of disease in the physical body and that the spirit is negatively affected before physical or emotional health is affected. (Gerber describes the etheric body as a part of the aura, the energy field that surrounds the physical body that can be seen in Kirlian photography.)

Trauma comes in many guises. These days we hear a lot of credence given to a chemical imbalance in the brain being the cause of mental illness. Too rarely is it understood that change in the chemical properties of the brain can be caused by trauma—a blow to the psyche, or a series of blows to the psyche. Usually there is no connection made between trauma and chemical imbalance. Although it can happen that a person is born with a chemical imbalance, or a predisposition to mental illness, a study of case histories of the mentally ill would lend credence to the hypothesis that the majority of those who are "mentally ill" or "emotionally disturbed" are plagued by the results of emotional injury— that the etheric body, the spirit, was affected first. When this is understood, the cure often becomes available, for it becomes a matter of treating the spirit, in an effort to reconstitute the healthy chemical constituents of the brain.

In her book *Talk Therapy,* psychiatrist Dr. Susan Vaughan writes in detail about how psychotherapy, like medication, changes the brain. But whereas medication can sometimes be toxic, psychotherapy works within a medium that is more natural. It works with a set of understandings toward a change in the belief system. Freud wrote extensively about psyche, in his native German. How the word "psyche" was translated varies from being called "soul" to "mind." Psyche governs the total organism, including the physical organism. A blow to the psyche can be more devastating than a blow to the physical body.

Modern medicine, which we would not want to do without, would benefit greatly by recognizing the emotional and spiritual components of health. Because the components of modern medicine and the components of holistic healing are largely based on attributes of the left and right hemispheres of the brain, respectively, often people going to see their family doctor do not mention that they might be getting help from acupuncture or hypnotism or Reiki. That is beginning to change, however. Even though some doctors refuse to recognize the benefits of "right-brain" healing, there is what might be called a grass roots movement going on. Insurance companies are beginning to recognize that it may be less expensive in the long run to start paying for some holistic modalities, as well as what has come to be called conventional medicine. And because money is equal to a kind of power, more doctors are pushed to recognize the possibility of changes in the medical horizon. Many professional groups are now sponsoring conferences on the dual topic of Science and Spirituality. A new paradigm is forming.

Werner Heisenberg, who is largely responsible for the revolution in physics known as quantum mechanics, is the father of the uncertainty principal, which has had profound philosophical implications. The idea that subatomic reality cannot be said to obey precise laws opens the door for the possibility of what could be called spirit in the bailiwick of Nature. This is a profound change which is only beginning to be fully understood. Now that science and spirituality are beginning to be co-sponsored, Heisenberg's hope for interesting developments to come from the interactions between different cultural environments begins to exist in the realm of reality.

A Medical Dichotomy
From Cooperation to Coercion

The National Center for Complementary and Alternative Medicine, a new Division of the National Institute of Health, was formed in order to help bridge the gap between the medical community and alternative treatments such as branches of Oriental medicine. It has given grants for research to medical schools including Columbia, Johns Hopkins and Harvard. Sizeable grants have been given to two small schools of alternative medicine as well. Each of those small schools is a school of acupuncture.

My first reaction to this idea was that finally the two schools of thought, one representing left brain thinking, the other right brain thinking, would be combined, thereby benefiting both schools. Obviously, whole brain thinking is involved with each school, but the thinking style which is emphasized is what makes for a dramatic difference. Whereas the medical model can be seen as technological in its means and in its understandings, it is representative of a tool, whereas branches of Oriental medicine can be considered as having more to do with spirit. The idea of bridging the gap between what can be considered left and right brain modalities is excellent. This could be considered the equivalent of a Corpus Callosum between medical models, an integrative technique that could benefit both schools of thought. But a representative of NCCAM says about acupuncturists in the supposed union of modalities: "It forces them (the acupuncturists) to start thinking about teaching the next generation of acupuncturists to think critically from a scientific perspective." This scientific representative of NCCAM wants acupuncturists to learn how to do scientific research.

Here is an age-old pattern, the pattern which may be what philosophers are talking about when they say we have taken a wrong turn in evolution. The tool, an invention, is telling spirit how to do things. How would the world be if spirit were telling tool how things should be done, rather than tool telling spirit? In other words, why is the medical model not wondering more why acupuncture is able to accomplish what it does rather than trying to push acupuncture into the scientific medical model?

If the medical model begins to prescribe to the model which incorporates acupuncture, is there not a threat of killing the goose that can lay golden eggs, of taking away the freedom of transcendence that spirit knows how to do, of killing the heartbeat of years of the growth of intuitive knowledge? Rather than trying to "force" acupuncturists to think scientifically, perhaps a better way to proceed with this supposed bridge would be for the scientists to learn acupuncture, and let them then apply their scientific rules, which would then be influenced by the fluctuating rules of the individual spirit. Perhaps the old adage of "if it isn't broken, don't try to fix it," may apply here. We may be in danger of making a tool turn into a wrecking ball.

A COOPERATIVE
CORPUS CALLOSUM
Drawing on Both Sides of the Brain

David Servan-Schreiber's book *The Instinct to Heal. Curing Stress, Anxiety, and Depression without Drugs and without Talk Therapy* is as good an example as one will get about the importance of the left brain supporting right brain attributes, hopefully the way the Corpus Callosum will best be used in our future. Call it complementary medicine or alternative medicine, the treatment methods that could be classified as either of these would be considered more the gifts of the right hemisphere than of the left, given how the characteristics of each have been classified.

And so the news from a psychiatrist is notable. Trained in the medical model, Servan-Schreiber was one of the legions of doctors who had learned to give medication as a front-line method of treatment. Then he began to see that more natural methods of healing, such as meditation and acupuncture, could deal with more of a cure, whereas medication was more of a possible cure for <u>symptoms.</u> Because he was thinking "outside of the box," his colleagues tended to deride his unconventional means of psychiatric help. Knowing both sides of the treatment modalities, Servan-Schreiber set out to prove scientifically that the cures of "the emotional brain" were not only beneficial, but tended to be curative rather than just giving symptomatic relief. Fortunately, this doctor had the left brain ability to tap into scientific mediums to support healing modalities that were the outgrowth of what could be seen as right hemisphere endeavors.

Rather than using the terms "left vs. right hemisphere," Servan-Schreiber uses the terms "cognitive vs. emotional brains." Because recent understandings have led toward the belief that the right hemisphere is a significant gateway to the limbic system, the emotional brain Servan-Schreiber talks about represents the right half of the Neocortex, sometimes cooperating with the cognitive, left hemisphere, sometimes silently in competition with its closely connected partner. Servan-Schreiber's ability to transcend (not to discard) his training makes him a champion of right brain interests. Does he still prescribe medication? Yes, but whereas the majority of psychiatrists feel forced to depend more on medication than any other single modality because of time and financial constraints, Servan-Schreiber uses medication as just one tool in an enlarged field of treatment possibilities. His approach to treatment speaks to an unfortunate application of disciplinary constraints.

Anthropologist T. M. Luhrman did an exhaustive study on the psychiatric community, examining in detail what some lay persons as well as professional mental health workers have suspected, that in the development of the series of DSM catalogues something has gone very wrong, and that perhaps diagnosis is not as important as understanding the patient. In pointing this out she walks that line that is between being a visionary and being a proponent of a common sense approach.

Sometimes professionals as well as lay persons bridle whenever they hear someone referred to as a diagnosis. "He's a schizophrenic," or "She's a borderline." In some opinions, he is Joe, and she is Mary, and each has a certain set of problems. It may very well be that through healing modalities of what can be considered the right hemisphere that Joe and Mary can be helped to cure their hurt by learning to know themselves rather than having their feelings put on ice with medication.

CREATIVITY AND PSYCHOPATHOLOGY
Strange Works of Art

Rollo May has made an important distinction between the ideas encapsulated in the words "demonic" and "daemonic." Whereas "demonic" is seen as evil, "daemonic" represents an energy which is Janus-like, of two faces, including a positive creative force. The symbolism evidenced in the symptoms of the mentally ill is an example of the creative forces inherent in the daemonic. The symptoms are the attempt to "fix" what is wrong. Just as an artist attempts to give form to an idea, a neurotic or a psychotic does the same. A successful work of art reflects a universal meaning, and even though the creation of the neurotic or psychotic is meaningful to that person alone, even though the symbolism is not consciously understood, the intent is the same, that is, to give form to an idea, in this case an idea to somehow undo the cause of the illness. Very rarely is this an efficient means of dealing with the problem, but this does not make the attempt any less imaginative. Not being able to remember an event that has been traumatic to a child is in one way an efficient way of dealing with something "too painful to remember." The ensuing anxiety, however, is a high price to pay for the sort of immunity that is afforded.

More and more it becomes apparent that there is a relationship between the symptoms of the mentally ill and what can be seen as a form of artistic creation. It is provocative to think that aberrant behavior is in its own way the attempt to "fix" what is wrong. There is a general axiom dictating that in order to prosper, one would do well to fit into the social realm of which one is a part, even if it is not a healthy environment. Artists tend to exemplify understandings that precede a general understanding. When society gives mixed messages, some are easily put off balance—perhaps the most sensitive, or perhaps those with a poor support system.

Modern art and modern music reflect a vibrant awareness of the chaos enveloping the planet on an unprecedented scale. Some bizarre attitudes are shaping the fabric of our lives, and in the ensuing chaos it is no coincidence that crimes are being committed in high places. Art embodies meaning, and the artists and the neurotic/psychotic have in common that they live from the unconscious depths of the society. They exemplify understandings that precede general understanding. The self-inflicted cuts on an incest survivor's body give meaning more immediate than we may want to bear witness to. These people are barometers of society. The symptoms are a key to the unconscious defense system, a kind of depth perception to the mind. When one considers that it has only been within the past century that the idea of an inner reality was even accepted, terms such as "mind exploration," now popularly accepted, are still somewhat revolutionary. Just as Martha Graham tried to make manifest the spirit of Jung's Collective Unconscious in dance, there is a spirit in the cutters and burners that is a testament to the daemonic trying to make manifest the insensitivity of a powerful and sadistic force in society, revealing a monumental fury in one way, and symbolizing a collective martyrdom in another. It is devastating to see victims denying what has been done to them by the people they love, for fear of losing the people they love. Many will doubt their own sanity before they will acknowledge the deceit and betrayal of those on whom they have had to depend for nurturance. One of the lessons they have learned is that love can be a synonym for cruelty.

In phone sessions with one of these patients, let's call her Jill, who as a child was a victim of severe sexual, physical and psychological abuse, a therapist unconsciously tried to redirect Jill's suicidal feelings away from Jill herself. After many of the phone calls the therapist would find in her doodlings on her notepad a series of arrows doing a U-turn on the page, an obvious though unconscious attempt to cure Jill's suicidal depression and somatic symptoms by rerouting the feelings of victimization and helplessness onto the more appropriate avenue of acknowledging another set of feelings toward her perpetrators.

There now appears to be a kind of Collective Unconscious of the wounded—a personal martyrdom that is expressing a psychic pain that demands redress. This strange new kind of artist, whose forebears perhaps were those who wore hair shirts and beat themselves with cat-o'-nine-tails, will not be denied its artistry. It may be that this new kind of artist is forging a changing emotional climate in the world before the world in general is aware. Like someone putting an ear to the ground to hear a train in the distance, the artistry of the self-hurters obeys a dictum not yet consciously understood. This, the artistry of the self-hurters, is the first step, spilling out the pain by focusing the rage on the self. It is not possible that the psychic structure can be rebuilt without understanding the source of the rage. It is no coincidence that part of getting better is when the victims begin to hear, "It is not your fault."

Although at times it seems that evil is going to take over the world, there is another possibility. It may be that we are in the throes of an evolutionary advance, not only in the discovery of but in the development and restructuring of that amorphous commodity which combines mind and feeling called the human spirit. With these mentally ill, the right brain conduit to the Unconscious has been functionally shut down; access has to be gained to the unwanted information which has been hidden in order for the wounded spirit to survive. In order to grow, the spirit demands redress. Naming how the spirit was wounded is a beginning.

There is an army of young people whose daemonic, powerfully energetic, helpless in all ways but one, is demanding of us, "DO SOMETHING!" Decades ago Havelock Ellis wrote, "..it is impossible to conceive of any impulse in a human heart which cannot be transformed into Truth or into Beauty or into Love." That, I believe, is what is being demanded by these "mentally ill," in a descant which is only beginning to be heard.

Echoes and Promises
Our Footprints on the Path of Evolution

We are but a dot on a graph depicting life on this planet from its beginning. In an evolutionary sense, humans are infants, and as a baby learns one skill at a time before developing other skills, we learned to use the body. Although the unconscious was there before what could be identified as "mind," modern society has tended to ignore the unconscious, instead harnessing the powers of the conscious mind. Only very recently have we begun to give respect to the subtle power evoked by the unconscious. Our tendency in this technological age is to leave a part of us out of our everyday functioning, and stress levels have become so high that illness is becoming pervasive. Now we look to our hidden powers. In a technological society people are pawns, and there is a growing tendency to begin to investigate powers that have been in hiding. In this essay, if not the hero, the individual is at least the protagonist.

When I was very young I had the idea that if everyone were to share his or her particular knowledge, the secrets of the universe would unfold. As I started growing up the idea was dismissed as being naive, yet it would not be abandoned.

The older I grew, and the more I grew, the more I believed that this idea had relevance. The belief has grown and has contrapuntally developed as my reading has taken me into segments of the world as seen through other eyes and other minds.

Because every brain is at least slightly different from every other brain, and because the field of vision and thus of perceptions differs with everyone, every mind's eye will see something at least slightly different from the person next to him or her. No single individual will always be right as to philosophical implications of what he or she is seeing. Only when there is an inter-visionary understanding can we begin to understand the answers to the most basic questions such as "What is the best way to do everything, and why?

The riddles of the universe will not be answered here, but perhaps some appropriate questions will at least be raised as to what makes for our survival and for our well-being. In their broader scope these questions concern the evolution of the human psyche. In a more limited sense they probe the individual's place in nature. Nuggets of thought from scientists, humanists, nature writers and religious and spiritual leaders make up the mosaic of ideas which should prove to be more than the sum total of the many-hued pieces that make up the collage of our understandings.

There has been a growing tendency to downplay the importance of the individual's influence on the quality of life, yet it is only with an ability to assess the quality of individual perceptions that we will be able to escape what has become a populace worse than what has been called "A Nation of Sheep." We are in danger of becoming a nation of lemmings, lemmings who at times of overpopulation join each other in a mass migration, rushing into the sea and extinction. Symbolically, we race for weapons capable of mass extinction. There is an illustrious company that maintains we do have choices, choices which metaphorically speaking may be as simple as learning to lead with the right hemisphere instead of the now-traditional left.

Metaphorically speaking, although we use both left and right, which leads—right or left—can make monumental differences in the quality of our lives. When we lead with the right (brain) we begin to see the dangers of blindly following leaders who in truth are only seeing the benefits to themselves. As early as 1973 *The American Connection* by John Pekkanen warned of the growing power of the drug companies, power that had to do with greed rather than with service to humanity. The drug companies have been devastatingly successful. In spite of the frightening list of possible side effects of psychopharmacological medicines, even general practitioners today freely prescribe these medications, apparently unaware that in doing so they are interfering with the individual's ability to self-heal. There appears to be not enough time for a personal relationship between physician and patient to make possible the hope of a cure of more than just the symptom.

There is beginning to be an understanding that each of us has the responsibility to get in touch with our own unique way of thinking, and thus of healing. When one considers, however, that we are being manipulated on all sides by corporate interests which have a great deal to lose by people thinking and feeling for themselves, we start to realize that the change in understanding is not happening fast enough, as we have become the most drug-oriented culture in the history of the world. We have been duped into being a nation of non-thinkers and non-feelers so that someone else can make a big profit. The irony is that one of the appeals behind this so-called ethical drug use is that drugs alter consciousness. We deteriorate when we should be growing.

Scientist Donald Carr speaks of the vulgarization of thought that has resulted from standardized thinking, making the mass mind less than the the sum of its parts, while it should be greater by far. It is our responsibility to determine what matters most to us, what we care about most, and to understand the importance we have as individuals. Sometimes this takes more courage than we have been given the understanding to think is appropriate. Erich Fromm spoke of "the pathology of normalcy." We are full of knowledge, and only just beginning to understand. Bits of knowledge are the pegs on which we hang the cloak of our understandings. Our attitudes and our understandings, although they cannot be seen, felt, smelled, heard or tasted in pure form, are the most real things in our lives. They are the shapers of our selves and our world. We carry the seed of our evolution as human beings within us.

Philosopher Susanne Langer in one of her many books pointed out that the individual life shows in microcosm the pattern of human evolution. Leonard Shlain in his revelatory tome *The Alphabet Versus the Goddess* investigates the mystery of why matriarchal societies disappeared, "changing the sex of God," as he put it. How we are, what we do, changes the direction of our evolution.

Rupert Sheldrake points out that when nature develops a new pattern that it is easier for others to follow suit, so that philosophically speaking, nature has a memory. Taking the first step to individualized thinking makes the ongoing creativity of individual thought more of a possibility. The poet May Sarton thought to be able to see things "with a naked eye" was the mark of a genius. Easy it is not, but we have been given the gifts of many aptitudes. Which aptitudes we choose to develop will determine how we grow as a people, or how we will destroy whatever we touch.

A TALE OF TWO CATS
Animal Intuition

I have a funny story to tell you, a story that in some ways resembles a fairy tale. Once upon a time there was a young woman who had two cats, neither of whom purred or meowed. The young woman was a patient of mine, and this is the story she told me. At first she had not known of the significance of the quietness of her cats. She had only known that her cats had never purred, and that all of a sudden they purred, a lot. Myra (let's call her Myra) said that she noticed that both cats started to purr at just about the same time. Did one start to purr and then the other caught on, or was it more a matter of their both being ready to purr at the same time?

The only thing she could think of was that she had started telling people that she was going to be leaving a job soon, a job which often caused her blood pressure to go up to alarming heights. The company nurses seemed to take it more seriously than Myra did, but Myra knew she just didn't feel good at such times, as though her head might explode. So maybe the cats heard her talking about getting away from a toxic environment and understood, or that they were picking up on the elevated mood that was engendered when Myra thought about getting away from the toxic environment.

Myra's story continued: At one point she had been given a couple of Reiki treatments by a sympathetic friend. Her blood pressure was somewhat improved, and that was marvelous. Although she had a heightened appreciation for what she considered to be a right-brain healing modality, she thought no more about it.

Then one day she heard her friend, the one who had given her the Reiki treatments, telling someone else about Reiki, saying that it was good for all kinds of cures and/or damage control, and mentioned how animals also could benefit from this kind of treatment, as well as humans, and that animals are especially sensitive to Reiki. Myra said that although she didn't remember dreams, she often woke up in the morning knowing something she hadn't known when she went to bed the previous night. The day after Myra heard this about animals and Reiki she woke up, and in that hypnopompic state between sleep and wakefulness she realized that the two cats had begun purring just about the time she had been given her two Reiki treatments.

This had been a startling realization. The cats had not had a Reiki treatment, but apparently were responding to a change in her from her treatment. All Myra remembered at that point was that the Reiki person had done something like a quiet scan of her body, not even touching her most of the time. At the end of the second treatment, the Reiki person had commented that Myra's broken heart had been able to mend itself. Myra said that she wept when she heard that because she felt it was true. Just as someone cries as though in anguish only when the anguish has subsided, so it was with her. An incredulous Myra told me that somehow the cats must have been aware—that somehow they knew, that the cats must have been affected by a heaviness in the environment created by what had been her constant state of mourning. From what Myra had told me about happenings in her life, feelings of great loss should not have been unexpected.

Realizing that the cats had picked up on what had been her cure, that their intuitive sense seemed almost magical, Myra went on to say that she was reminded of a film she had seen at a conference on the subject of Science and Spirituality. Rupert Sheldrake, an English biochemist who had done extensive research on animal ESP, showed a film in which both a dog and the dog's owner, twenty miles apart, are filmed at the same time.

The dog is seen sleeping as the young woman to whom the dog belongs goes about her travels, lunching with a friend, then walking in the park. The two films share a split screen, one film of the sleeping dog, the other film centered on the dog's mistress. As the dog sleeps, the dog's mistress is seen sharing a park bench with her friend. Then, after the young woman tells her friend it is time she headed for home, then getting up from the park bench to go toward her car, the dog is seen continuing to sleep for a minute or so, and then getting up and slowly going toward the door, where he sits and looks out the screen door. Was this coincidence? Or did the dog pick up his owner's intention, even though she was twenty miles away?

Myra felt that the cats had helped her to a new recognition of the bond between animals and humans. The cats had recognized that she was feeling better, and Myra said it was probably before she realized that she was feeling better. The knowledge that the cats' "state of mind" had taken on a new dimension because her own spirit had been buoyed up was amazing to her. At first Myra had thought that she was feeling better because the cats had started to purr. But with the realization that the cats were responding to a change in her made it clear to Myra that we tend to overlook the exquisite gift of intuitive knowledge that animals possess.

Laughing, Myra said that what happened after that must have been a second wonderful surprise, for the cats. She said that she had been so grateful that these two little cats were so tuned into her that in place of the chunk tuna fish which had been their main diet that she had started feeding them solid white. (Until she discovered the high mercury content—then she switched to more chicken, and a combination of egg, rice and cheese.)

ERSATZ SCHIZOPHRENIA
An Iatrogenic Medical Model

A way of treating mental illness that is counterproductive has come to be taken for granted in many avenues of our society. Perpetuated by the arbitrary nature of the *Diagnostic and Statistical Manual of Mental Disorders,* published by the American Psychiatric Association, diagnosis is not consistently reliable. In most public health agencies there is heavy use of the "Schizophrenia" diagnosis. As Peter Kramer acknowledges in his book *Listening to Prozac,* "Considering diagnosis a mere administrative requirement, American psychiatrists (have begun) calling all seriously ill patients schizophrenic."

Because treatment for the mentally ill is largely in the hands of psychiatrists, the drug companies and the insurance companies, an individual with a "mental problem" is compromised. The insurance companies will not pay for treatment without a diagnosis. After the diagnosis, in most cases medication is the first line of treatment. Behavior modification may be a possible corollary. Both of these forms of treatment attempt to control symptoms, rather than to investigate and then to work through to an understanding of the cause of the illness. This insures long-term treatment, as medication causes its own problems, and the disease itself is only masked by medications.

The main focus of psychiatric day treatment facilities has been to try to keep patients out of the hospital. A very small percentage of these clients have had psychotherapy, and even fewer are not on psychotropic medication. The popular culture has little problem with the concept of trying to fix everything with a pill. By consistently treating the symptoms and neglecting the causes, a direct connection is established between the large number of people who remain "severely and persistently mentally ill," even though "a quick fix" is what was intended. Why, in such a highly educated group of professionals, is more credence not given to getting to the root of problems? The answer is not far away. "Quicker" is considered a saving of time—and money. As it is there is a shocking lack of recognition that repressed feelings are toxic agents causing illness. Until these feelings are dealt with, the illness does not go away, it just gets repressed, pushed down into the realms of the Unconscious. The necessity of working through feelings is overlooked, and psychotropic medication helps the patient to retreat even further from the feelings whose denial has caused the illness.

When a person, especially a child, is neglected and abused, shame and humiliation can be compounded into suicidal and homicidal feelings, or be translated into delusions and hallucinations. It is not difficult for a profound reservoir of hurt and shame to be translated into latent anger. As a society we do not know how to deal with anger, and for this we pay a terrible price. Seldom is it heard from one of the legions of the mentally ill that it is all right to be angry. Typical comments when asked about anger are, "Anger is dangerous." Or "Bad things happen when people get angry." Or, "It isn't a good idea to feel anger." For the most part anger is feared. When anger is denied, squelched, projected and otherwise deflected, by the time it insists on expression it becomes so explosive that psychiatric hospitalization and psychotropic medication seem expedient.

Feelings need to be acknowledged. Feelings of hurt and humiliation, relegated to the dark and silent interior of the mind, ferment until bizarre aberrations and a quiet rage take the place of healthy development. Abraham Maslow put it very well: "Every crime against our nature records itself in our Unconscious and makes us despise ourselves." Voices prohibited in reality are internalized, free to issue condemnations toward self and toward others.

People are betrayed by the words "chemical imbalance." While it is possible that a newborn can have a predisposition toward chemical imbalance, it is more probable that a chemical imbalance of the brain has been caused by an inability to cope with a hostile environment. The body and mind are so closely bound together that mental anguish can cause chemical changes in the brain. It further complicates the situation that when a diagnosis is in question that psychiatrists often use "schizophrenia" as a catchall diagnosis. Depression and anxiety are relatively easier to diagnose, but if delusions or hallucinations are present, the illness is seen as psychosis, and schizophrenia is an easy jump from there. Once a patient is diagnosed as schizophrenic chances are that patient will be on psychotropic medication for the rest of his or her life—the patient becomes the illness. And the drug companies have one more notch in the ever increasing size of their money belts. In *Your Drug May Be Your Problem,* Peter Breggin, M.D. and David Cohen, Ph.D. explore the danger to the human spirit inherent in the cavalier and overzealous prescribing of psychotropic medications. Both body and mind have healing capacities that are compromised by what is simply part of a system of control, rather than a healing modality.

One of the patients whom I would identify as having an "ersatz schizophrenia" diagnosis recently told me that his schizophrenia is in remission. Now, rather than paying attention to his inner resources for growth, he is attuned to whether he is "active" or not. As a child this man had been abused physically, emotionally and sexually. There was no support or understanding in the environment. Feelings were truncated, guilt ran rampant. ("If only I weren't so bad, this would not be happening") Eventually the feelings came out in hallucinations and paranoia, in his case aided and abetted by both drugs and alcohol.

Often feelings engendered by neglect and abuse do lead to substance abuse as a form of self-medication, to keep the emotional pain of the abuse from being felt. When attempts are made to drown out the humiliation and anger and the attendant anxiety that comes with all the feelings, the brain becomes chemically charged, especially with the toxicity of drugs and/or alcohol. Even though the DSM clearly states that hallucinations and delusions should not be drug related for the schizophrenic diagnosis, this directive is often overlooked. The client becomes twice damned. "Double trouble" is one name for it. MICA (Mentally ill chemical abusers) is another.

The dual diagnosis can tag a person for life. The distinction is not made that the voices, hallucinations or delusions may be from the chemical changes elicited by both emotional and substance abuse. Even though the patient may become clean and sober, and be able to deal effectively with some of the emotional residue, the mental illness label often becomes a permanent fixture in the person's life. The patient, in effect, becomes his illness, and loses the capacity for change and growth. The illness becomes part of the paperwork, copied onto new records year after year. And the patient often remains a mentally ill statistic, someone who feels there is no exit.

When the personal dynamic of growth is arrested it cannot proceed until the tangle of feelings has been uncovered and processed. Psychotropic meds make cure more difficult by just covering up the symptoms and dulling the curative forces that are part of our biological equipment. From dreams to the detective work of free association, talk therapy can be used to gradually give victims back their integrity, replacing the stultifying effects of the psychopharmacological tools. Respect and empathy for the victim give dignity to the individual, rather than to the illness. This tends to treat the root system of the problem rather than just the symptoms, becoming a restorative technique to offset the chemical imbalance caused by the trauma of abuse. Susan Vaughan, M.D., states unequivocally in *The Talking Cure: The Science Behind Psychiatry,* that talk therapy changes the chemistry of the brain, toward restoring and improving normal functioning.

Because control is so powerfully vested in the business of mental illness, it is probable that any change is going to be the result of a grass roots movement. It does not appear that the *Diagnostic and Statistical Manual of Mental Disorders* is going out of style. According to *Making Us Crazy**, a *DSM-V is* in preparation. But what if we could come up with a diagnosis that would make an exit from "the system" more possible? What if we were to come up with a different category for future Diagnostic and Statistical Manuals? What if we were to establish a category "UFS: for "Unidentified Feeling Syndrome?" This would change the attitude toward illnesses that do not fit neatly into one of the categories already established, such as schizophrenia, and would acknowledge the importance of emotional components that have a better chance of being "fixed." An attitude of keeping mental illness under control would be

---

* By Herb Kutchins and Stuart Kirk. Subtitle: "*DSM: The Psychiatric Bible and the Creation of Mental Disorders.*"

transformed into the idea of searching the psyche for traces of a sensitivity to abuse. The individual could be treated as a unique entity whose reactive behaviors emerged from his or her personal history.

Rachel Carson, who long ago recognized that we are killing Nature with our man-made pesticides pointed out that whenever we substitute something man-made and artificial for something natural that we retard part of a person's spiritual growth. What has happened with so many of our Seriously and Persistently Mentally Ill is that their spiritual growth has been dwarfed by the ingestion of man-made medicines, the purpose of which is to keep feelings, also known as symptoms, under control. Thus the positive natural healing possibilities of human nature are prevented from evolving.

It all comes down to an attitude. Those who have control over the lives of so many of the mentally ill may not be seeing the whole picture. Are we willing to cooperate with Nature, including the self-healing possibilities of human nature, or must we insist on controlling Nature, even though we are killing what we claim to love the most?

THE DARK HORSE
Dream, Out of Right Brain

Sometimes feelings get shunted off behind some kind of a closed door, and dreams can be an important tool of discovery. Dreams give us pictures of our feelings, and as we learn to decipher our dream language we gain insights which make our lives more understandable.

Without feeling, thinking has no root system, and tends to be superficial. Without thought, feelings can be overwhelming. Once we are in touch with how we feel, we need to know what we want to do with the feelings. Integrating thought and feeling is one of the more delicate tasks of the human brain, which has so many working parts that more than one brain expert has called the brain *terrifyingly* complex. It is now common knowledge that the two hemispheres of the cerebrum, or neo-cortex, connected by a large band of fibers called the corpus callosum, represent separate and distinct styles of thinking.

Individual differences are noticed in the fetal brain; each of us is born different from anyone else. Then, along with physiological differences, the brain grows and changes according to environment. In the fetus, the right hemisphere develops before the left, which supports the hypothesis that the right hemisphere came first evolutionarily. There is also evidence that the left hemisphere was developed as a tool. Ninety-five percent of the population has the language center in the left hemisphere, and language is an efficient tool. But it may be that the wisdom of the right brain has been sacrificed.

In our culture the left hemisphere is in charge, while the right hemisphere many times has difficulty saying what it sees. The left hemisphere has been called the praxic brain, implying that it is the brain that does things, the brain that keeps things in order, the brain that in many ways is like a digital-type computer. The right hemisphere has been called the gnosic brain, suggesting superior wisdom and knowledge of mystical and spiritual truth. But what if the right brain is considered inconsequential? Carl Jung, the most famous of all psychoanalysts save Freud, pointed out that the gifts of the head and heart are seldom found in the same person. This is where the great paradox comes in. Although right brain thinking is regarded as the keeper of the sense of values, our society is based on left-brain thinking. What the right brain does has been so difficult to classify that what it does has come to not be considered thinking at all.

Based on research data, some theorists think that the left hemisphere behaves like a competitive individual, an independent mind that inhibits its partner. Because it is the right hemisphere that sees the whole picture, important nuances, feelings and understandings often remain unarticulated and/or cut down by its competitive skull mate. And when the competitor skull mate, the left brain, talks about a system of values, chances are that values are being specified which have more to do with self-interest than the good of the many.

We learn how to see things as we grow up; we learn <u>what</u> to think. The dream, a right-brain activity, can help us learn <u>how</u> to think by helping us to better know our feelings. Out of dysfunctional families and our image-conscious society, many a false self has been created. The wisdom of the dream can help us to become more real. Understanding of the dream, <u>which must be interpreted by the linguistic left hemisphere</u> can help to make us whole. Although Freud has called the dream the Royal Road to the Unconscious, the Corpus Callosum, that large band of connecting fibers between the hemispheres, may be the road to understanding the dream, and thus our feelings.

A few years ago a study was done on dreams according to hemisphere preference of the dreamers which found that while right-brainers remembered more dreams and had more metaphorical dreams than left-brainers, attitude toward dreams made a difference, even with left-brainers. Even among those with left-brain preference, those who had more respect for the significance of the process of dreaming remembered more dreams and had a broader range of symbolism.

It seems that the beginnings of consciousness may have begun with the dream. Perhaps by nudging the quarks of consciousness through our dream life we can build a new, less divisive, foundation of consciousness. Every dream can be considered a building block toward a fuller understanding of ourselves. Even the nightmare can be put to use if it is seen as the grout of primitive energy from which a mosaic of positive creative efforts can be spawned. As we begin to develop more confidence in the whole of us with the aid of such as the dream, perhaps the brain will begin to be understood as *wonderfully* complex. And our society will be less divisive the more that we understand the importance of the gifts of the dream and of the metaphorical right brain.

ON EDUCATION
Assembly-Line Learning

Standards are important. There can be no argument but that it is good to have standards. But when standards turn into standardized, that is not so good. In educational and professional tracks, when they who have the power to tell us what intellectual path we must take in order to be considered proficient enough to be considered educated, are these minds of ours in effect not being cloned to be like the minds under whose tutelage they are being educated? That the motive is not meant to be harmful does not alter the outcome of the learners' minds being pushed into cubicles. With too few exceptions, innovation is diluted by a mass-produced mind. What if the germ of some vital idea is sheared away in the process of making conceptions fit a mold? How is this not the same as putting one's mind in a box? Limiting potential, teaching what to think, rather than how to think, not only shows a lack of respect for individuality, but curtails ideas that have the possibility of solving some of our most enduring problems. This wonderful collective brain, having the ability to use individuality to shape evolution in a natural and meaningful way, "a self-organizing universe," becomes stuck in pre-ordained tracks. It is like asking the brain to do its best work on canned thoughts instead of the creative freshness of which some of the strongest minds are capable.

Science methodology, one of our inventions which has been "put in charge," mandates that individual thought is not considered "scientific." Yet the intuitions of our thinking may be the most valuable part of our intellectual system. To denigrate this part of our mental armamentarium is the equivalent of tying our hands and feet together and telling us to run.

It is the intuitive right hemisphere, seeing the whole picture, which has the ability to come up with some of our most productive solutions to our problems. Although the right hemisphere develops first in the fetus, it is thought that both hemispheres are very much the same at birth, with each hemisphere developing through a kind of training process. Although there is a necessity for the hemispheres to work together, one hemisphere, probably more through training than genetic endowment, will take charge. Because of the importance of verbal thinking in our society, most are nudged more toward the strong left-brain school than into the less highly-regarded right brain pool of thinkers. Our educational strengths have been focused on left-brain attributes, and non-verbal thinking has been relegated to being considered inferior, because words have come to be the measure of intelligence.

Lewis Terman, who developed the IQ test, believed that reasoning with verbal concepts is the highest expression of intelligence. This has set a standard for our society which has undermined the spiritual, the artistic and the intuitive, and perhaps most important of all has pushed aside the attitude that values cooperation above competition. Values themselves are the escutcheon of the right hemisphere. Until recently values have not been considered an important consideration in the field of science, in the halls of think tanks, or in the educational classroom. And, in a society which does not value values, it comes as no surprise that there is a whole lot of cheating going on, from SAT testing to white collar criminality on Wall Street.

Occasionally the complaint is heard that creative thinkers and artists are becoming more rare in the population. How could it be otherwise? Whereas there used to be educational alternatives between farm, shop, apprenticeship or even individual tutoring, now school is demanded for everyone, making individual aptitudes less meaningful, and turning schools into what at times seems more like a penal system than a place of learning. An ignorance of the "unconscious" side of the brain is coupled with a disregard for our intuitive gifts. An understanding of the importance of an educated instinct tends to be relegated to mothers, entrepreneurs and the unemployed.

The world of academia at times is taken over by a world in which left-brain thinkers admire each other's left-brain work, with Ph.D. students becoming entrenched in left-brain thinking, forfeiting the intuitive and creative gifts of their metaphorical right brain. When this happens the left-brain system of thinking perpetuates itself. There are times when highly intuitive people are in danger of trading in some of their gifts for the book learning that is the basis of a graduate degree. This is why our "whole-brain" thinkers are so valuable. And why they often have to step outside the fragmented disciplines of learning. Right brain skills are not able to be part of committee thinking because it is difficult for the right brain to read, write or talk, which is why one person can sometimes be more efficient than a committee.

An appropriate analogy for this can be found in an observation from a situation concerning the large number of homeless in New York City. Because of the large homeless population, with many families living out of cardboard boxes, a consortium was held to see what could be done to help to improve the situation. It was thought to be a good idea to delegate a group of city officials and representatives from social and political agencies to work on the problem. Not one of those in the group was from the cadre of the homeless. Who better would <u>know</u> the problems, and perhaps be able to suggest remediation?

As intellectual qualities are stressed, values, which establish the attitude out of which organization grows, sometimes tend to be overlooked or used to promote individual interests. Intellectual training sometimes tends to destroy the quality of intuition. A danger is that the attitude of professionals who have been educated to "fit" may work in their professional lives with an eye toward helping those whom they train to "fit" rather than to help them to draw upon their own self-actualizing techniques and individualistic modes of growth. When one is made to fit a model, the tendency will be toward helping "the other" to fit a model. Decades ago muckraker Lincoln Steffens noted that "the best ideas haven't been thought of yet."

When there is a strongly entrenched model for education and certification there is the encouragement to rehash old ideas. That is not to say that new ideas cannot be spawned from this mode, but the tendency is to get stuck in the tracks that have been laid down. Anything that does not first fit into these tracks may be seen as nothing more than an anachronism. Whether in science, medicine, education, or in psychotherapy, new ideas are often labeled as dangerous. Perhaps it is no coincidence that among brain researchers, neurosurgeons, and experimental psychologists, some report that the strong left hemisphere not only dominates its right hemisphere, but tends to regard its right hemisphere as inferior.

However, there are changes appearing on the horizon which are heartening. Alternative medicine is happening.

The various disciplines rising out of energy medicine are gaining in importance. Science is recognizing spirit. Some in the scientific community are recognizing that just because something can't be seen, tasted or smelled doesn't mean it isn't real, and this in itself is shaking up our old belief systems. Old values which have emphasized monetary and materialistic goals are being questioned. And a growing understanding of hemispheric differences is giving right brainers a new respect for what they know, thus establishing a paradigm that is resonating into every thinking discipline.

THE EMOTIONAL PALETTE
Shades of Meaning

"As the twig is bent, so grows the tree." This aphorism, generally used to describe the importance of the way a child is trained, also underlines the importance of habit. For the purpose of the discussion of the Emotional Palette we are talking about feelings that are learned very early, and for our purposes we are comparing these feelings to the various colors an artist might have on his or her palette, which would vary from one artist to another. The palette of emotions has to do with the assorted feelings generated by our individual environments from the time we are born, and perhaps even before.

There is an assumption that babies, unable to express their feelings in words, do not feel, or if they do feel that the feelings will not be remembered. On the contrary, pre~verbal feelings tend to be the most powerful because they cannot be named and thus worked with. But because that particular feeling path has been recorded in the brain, the feeling remains available even though the memory which set off the original feeling is not available. These original feelings, naturally come by, may be called on inappropriately simply because they are readily available. In the case of trauma, when memories are pushed into the Unconscious for a sort of cold storage, the old feelings often remain available, even when the original trauma is not consciously remembered.

An experiment conducted at the University of Wisconsin shows that abused children are extraordinarily sensitive to signs of anger in facial expressions. Abuse victims were much quicker to see either fear or sadness as anger. Apparently, tracking the possibility of anger had become so important that they tended to see it where others did not, thus assuming nonexistent threats. *{Harvard Mental Health Letter,* May, 2003.)

As the memorization of a verse becomes more readily available the more it is practiced, so it can be with feelings. The more a certain feeling is aroused, the more available it is on the palette of available emotions. The more trauma a child is subjected to, the more sensitive the child will be to trauma, even though the memories of the trauma may not be available. When a strong feeling is learned, that feeling is apt to be depended on, especially in times of crisis. It might be compared with a path worn down through a field or meadow. Once traversed, it is easier to walk the same way again, rather than striking out on an unidentified route. The more that path is used, the more apt the traveler is to use that path. So it is with the pathways of feeling. Even though the original memories which have inspired the feeling may be unavailable, familiar feelings are relied on, and the feeling pathways become more entrenched.

Even with adults, painful memories are often shoved into the Unconscious. This is where our right brain gets us in trouble, for with its close connection to the Unconscious, the memory can easily be segued in that direction instead of hopping across to the left hemisphere to use its ability to put things into words. Without the skills of the left hemisphere the memories tend to be unavailable. One of the doctors who worked with survivors of horrendous multiple abuses commented about the most severely traumatized client he had ever seen, let's call her Erica. He said, "If Erica could get on the radio and tell everything that happened, she would be cured." Erica had a diagnosis of Multiple Personality Disorder, now more commonly called Dissociative Identity Disorder.

Talking is a tool which can help in what is like an archaeological dig in the detective work of therapy. Just as the chemistry of the brain has been changed by trauma, putting darker colors on the emotional palette, putting feelings together with the memories which inspired those feelings will add a new feeling, a new color to the palette. And the chemistry of the brain once again is altered, in a way that siphons off some of the toxicity that has been the result of toxic experiences. Feelings of being understood, feelings of hope, feelings of self confidence begin to take on colors to add to the otherwise limited array of colors on the emotional palette. New pathways are established through the brain's field of neurological possibility.

As an adjunct to talk therapy, play therapy has established itself as a rewarding medium in working with both children and adults, especially if traumatization happened before the child had the use of speech. Especially from pre-verbal times, the effects of that abuse can be difficult to work through, and play therapy is a good way of eliciting ideas from pre-verbal times. I am especially reminded here of a young woman we'll call Melanie, who had been the victim of severe abuse as a small child. She was very intelligent, and very, very sad. With Melanie, play therapy proved its worth, adding brighter colors to her emotional palette. Sand play was the vehicle—words were not necessary. In the tray of sand new harbingers of strength were being played out, and new feelings learned and remembered. Sometimes metaphor becomes more available through a process of play. The thought of Melanie's joyful energy, unavailable to her until she was able to claim her strengths through the take charge attitude she displayed in the artistry of the sand tray, reminds me to this day of bells and whistles. If one were to know some of the sordid details of her childhood, that positive energy would seem to be miraculous.

Body therapy, too, has its place in mitigating the effects of the darkest colors on the palette, by siphoning off the toxic elements that the body remembers, even though the mind may not remember. *The Molecules of Emotion* by Dr. Candace Pert pictures the body as a complex repository of an aggregate number of little brains, each with its own set of emotions. Feelings inspired by trauma can get locked into various parts of the body, and then be freed by body work such as massage or Reiki. Then, when the person learns that he or she has been able to surmount what has seemed to be a constant state of emergency, a feeling of capability is introduced to the emotional palette. The capable feeling becomes available. The more the feeling is incorporated into the daily tapestry of emotion, the more helpful it becomes, and the more the individual is able to understand the meaning of Camus' "In the midst of winter, I finally learned that there was in me an invincible summer."

In addition to talk therapy, play therapy, and body therapy, there is another way of adding new colors to the emotional palette. Artistic endeavor—whether painting, music, dance, writing, or sculpture—uses unexpressed feelings to manufacture an artistic creation, transforming trauma into a celebratory transcendence. While childhood joy will tend to perpetuate itself into adulthood, Adult Children of Alcoholics (ACOA) maintain, "It is never too late to have a happy childhood."

Fundamental Values
Emotional and Social Astuteness

Rumor has it that President Eisenhower walked into a room full of computers and was told he could ask Univac any question he wanted. The then President allegedly typed into the keyboard, "Is there a God?" The story continues that after a short interval of whirring and buzzing a paper rolled out of the computer on which there were three words typed in capital letters, the first word underlined, "<u>NOW</u> THERE IS!" What has happened since then is history. With the advent of the computer the suggestion announces itself that God is more machine than spirit. Ergo, if there is an attitude that God is more machine than spirit, and if we believe that we are made in God's image, that would indeed make us more machine than spirit.

Ever more efficient technologically, modern medicine has adopted the philosophy of technology, treating the body and the mind as different parts of a machine— the human machine. The technology has become a system of measurements and a system of adding something or taking something away to fix a problem, physical or mental. Often strong feelings tend to be distrusted, rather than seen as signals to encourage soul searching. In the mental health field the concept of "The Broken Brain" takes hold, and when the brain is considered broken, there is the acceptance of the idea of a chemical imbalance which must be fixed by the ingestion of chemicals, a technological procedure, or even surgery, to counteract the chemical imbalance which has been the result of "the broken brain."

Psychopharmacology, along with biological psychiatry, has ruled the ever-widening arena of mental illness. The idea of the quick fix has established itself in psychiatry, and a pyramid of treatment has grown up from an industry which has taken control of a situation wherein people feel they are incapable of dealing with what they begin to see as "a chemical imbalance." The quick fix, however, turns out to be a try at the alleviation of symptoms. A temporary fix is far from a cure. Often a lifetime of medication with the resultant blunting of natural feelings is the result, this rather than an attempt to get at the root of what was the original cause of the problem, thus giving the possibility of a cure.

There are some schools of thought which differentiate themselves from the psychiatric modality in that they base their belief on the ability of the individual to tap into his or her own physical, spiritual and emotional resources to grow toward self-healing. The ability to trust such an empathic professional can treat more than symptoms. When only the symptoms are treated, the number of "Seriously and Persistently Mentally Ill" continues to grow. Although the dis-ease may be temporarily eased by the ingestion of pills, normal feelings are blunted, and the person's innate capacity to self-heal becomes less available, just when this capacity is needed most. Other therapies, however, take more time than writing out prescriptions. It takes a relatively short time to diagnose, to write out a prescription, and to prescribe again, and again, and again, all of this to keep symptoms, which have to do with feelings, under control. The illness, not the patient, becomes the star. Following the diagnosis comes the inevitable prescription for psychotropic medication. One of the many recovered who "used to believe in the biological model of mental illness" before his diagnosis of schizophrenia pointed out that feelings and dreams cannot be analyzed under a microscope and that recovery is facilitated by people who believe in you, who give you hope, and who understand your feelings.

Too seldom are dreams seen as therapeutic tools to help a person self-heal. A dream is a picture of a feeling. As medication blunts daytime feelings, it also thwarts dream activity. Trying to do a dream group in a treatment program for the mentally ill is like giving some really nutritious raw vegetables to people without teeth. The Unconscious has many answers for us if we can gain entry, and dreams are one door, or as Freud put it, a "royal road" to that special place. Dreams, talk therapy, body work, all are natural empowerments, along with good food, exercise and sleep. It may be that psychotropic medication is one of the examples of man having gone too far in his goal of conquering Nature. There is not yet a wide acceptance of the possibility that Nature may be more curative than chemistry.

Anyone who has taken case histories of those who become the "Persistently and Seriously Mentally Ill" can find ample evidence that there has most often been an assault on spirit before mental illness took root. But spirit cannot be measured, so it is overlooked. Illnesses become the focus of healing techniques which at best are superficial and at their worst are an abrogation of the power of the human spirit.

If we ask ourselves what our fundamental values are would we acknowledge that we most admire our ability to take control? Or could we say that we value the ability of people to "self-actualize?" Perhaps there have been many wrong turns in evolution. The outcome has been to leave behind, to fend for itself on a little-traveled back road, the acknowledgement of a living spirit. It is time we took a detour off the scientific highway and brought vitalism, the belief in spirit, onto the main road.

Our penchant for trying to keep things under control is only one example of how the linear, explicit, sequential, concrete and goal-oriented attributes of the left hemisphere do us a disservice. Dr. R. Joseph, author of *The Right Brain and the Unconscious: Discovering the Stranger Within*, is tactful in discussing this disservice: "If the left brain maintains functional dominance at all times and relegates the right brain to second-class status, the person may be put at a tremendous disadvantage, as the right brain is so emotionally and socially astute whereas the left brain is not."

Perhaps it is not too late to remedy the course human evolution has adopted and put back into our lives the recognition of an elan vital which Henri Bergson recognized many decades ago, and which is defined in *Webster's Dictionary* as "..the vital impulse which is the substance of consciousness and nature."

FREUD DID NOT
GO FAR ENOUGH
A Third Phase of Sexual Development

If Freud were alive today, perhaps he himself would see three, rather than two phases of sexuality as put forth in his *Three Essays on the Theory of Sexuality*. In this, one of his many works on sexuality, he wrote: "The fact that the onset of sexual development in human beings occurs in two phases, i.e. that the development is interrupted by the period of latency, seemed to call for particular notice. This appears to be one of the necessary conditions of our aptitude for developing a higher civilization, but also of our tendency to neurosis. As far as we know, nothing analogous is to be found in man's animal relatives." (p. 139)

Morton Hunt in *The Universe Within* points out that there is a relatively small evolutionary remnant of prehistoric brain in the human being, and a very large evolutionary innovation of forebrain and uncommitted cortex available for higher mental processes. This is what makes us human. Our uncommitted area is ours to use as we see appropriate. How we use this uncommitted area of the cortex is of vital importance. Our priorities will determine how we choose to use this gift.

The aftermath of the climacteric has proverbially been seen as the period of decline. To continue to see this phase of life as nothing but a decline may lend itself to the philosophical nihilism affecting our planet. In the unfolding of evolution certain patterns become more and more apparent. Physicists are discovering that the physical world can be represented in fewer and fewer patterns. It is appropriate that this should also be true of the psychological world. Just as there is a seeming try for "order out of chaos" in the physical world, so there should be the same thrust in the world of the psyche, or spirit, whether one speaks in terms of the individual, or of humanity as a whole. The uncommitted territory of the forebrain is available for the creative effort that will make the difference between our annihilation or, as presaged by Susanne Langer, "a New Season of Civilization." The climacteric could well be seen as the corresponding interruption between phases as was the period of latency.

Early in the twentieth century Henri Bergson noted that species evolve during individual lifetimes. Now our life expectancy is decades longer than it was a century ago. This, coupled with a burgeoning interest in the existence of "spirit", creates the possibility of a new paradigm which has implications for the scientific community. Even science, that stubborn holdout for "if you can't see it, it isn't real" is beginning to do research which proves that there are energies which are real, even though they cannot be measured in size or weight. The climacteric, a third phase of sexuality, is an appropriate arena for the recognition of the spiritual component of humanity, at the same time as the physical body recedes in strength.

The mathematician-philosopher Susanne Langer is just one of many who has suggested that we took "a wrong turn in evolution." She suggests that as a species we chose the path of what today might be called the world of the left hemisphere; that we tended to ignore a birthright which should have included a more feeling, intuitive, spiritual stance—more of the qualities attributed to the right brain. Donald Carr's *The Forgotten Senses* claims that we still have the ability for the kind of intuitive gifts that animals have, that these gifts have been glossed over for the world of measurement, language, and digital time, but that we are phylogenetically young enough to reclaim our intuitive heritage.

How we use our longer lifespan is up to us. If we see our lives in terms of a decline, then decline we shall. Because the average lifespan in Freud's time was decades shorter, he could not see the possibility of what the third sexual period in the life of humans could represent. As latency was the period between childhood sexuality and adult sexuality, the climacteric could represent the period between adult sexuality and the sublimation of sexuality representing a different kind of creative energy, toward using the wisdom of our years into the building of a set of understandings that will make a more viable set of life systems. Perhaps it is our choice whether to move toward more neurosis or toward a higher level of civilization.

Our brain's uncommitted area in the cortex could set new standards. In Nature there is a universal trend to grow toward the light. The decline of the physical life in the individual could represent the positive growth of the human spirit, a natural occurrence if we can only allow Nature to have its way with us.

The Myth of the Mayfly

Ultra Adult vs. Senior Citizen

People are living longer today, possibly longer than ever before. Living longer can be a time when priority goes to senescence or to synthesis; to a recognition of waning powers, or to a synergy of wisdom. Attitude can make all the difference. We can see ourselves as becoming worn-out machines, or as becoming rich with feeling for the meaning of life as we consolidate what we have learned over a lifetime.

It is not known whether attitude influences thinking style, or the other way around, but it is evident that different people have different thinking styles. Lately scientists are declaring as news things that poets have known all along. For example, a leading newspaper recently ran an article announcing that neuroscientists are finding that the brain need not deteriorate with age, that the brain can develop well into old age. Also, the research of a well-known physicist concludes that the meanings we ascribe to things will affect evolution. Another physicist finds that the more we learn, the more we find that nature favors just a few patterns.

Lately we also hear that our old myths are no longer adequate, and that God is dead. Myth and belief go hand in hand. Technology ascends in importance as other belief systems founder. Money and machines, invented by us as tools for our convenience, have become the sponsors of the predominant belief system.

By connecting the concepts concerning ongoing brain plasticity, the effect of attitude on evolution, and Nature's parsimony with patterns, we can make a difference for ourselves now, and a difference in how we evolve as a species. To put us in this more important place, a place where who we are and what we believe will make a difference, we need not invent myths—we need only to discover. The symbols for new myths are waiting for us if we look closely enough at Nature's patterns.

A myth suitable for today coming from the patterns of Nature can be seen in the prototype of the mayfly Ephemera vulgate. This mayfly is an anomaly in nature because it has two distinct adult forms, the second mature form being the one which deposits the eggs. Taking into consideration that people today often have segmented lives, many retiring only to start a second career, there appears to be a pattern in the life of this mayfly that may help us shape a myth which will be a natural barrier to today's depersonalization. Perhaps it is an idea overdue to think in terms of a collective progeny of the mind, or spirit, coming out of our later years—a synthesis of wisdom appropriate to what might be called our Ultra Adult phase.

In our first adult phase we produce physical progeny; in the Ultra Adult phase, why not a progeny of the psyche? It is most appropriate that what philosophers look to as a New Season of Civilization should start with a new season of the individual.

Listen, dear grown-up children, to this myth of our possible progression through time. Miracles may be no more than extended patterns of natural phenomena, after all.

****

Once upon a time—long, long after the time that Pandora opened Epimetheus' box to let loose all the evils thereafter known to humankind—someone dreamed that the magic box still held a strange and wonderful creature which had remained hidden in the box even after Hope had made her appearance into the world.

In the dream the box was opened again, and an exotic-looking insect with three feelers extending from the tail area flew out on four pearly lacelike wings. It rose up in the air and made dizzy spirals after temporary bouts of balancing itself on nothing in the midst of everything, only to thrust itself up and away again, and again, and again.

For all its darting about it seemed to the dreamer, who somehow in the dream had become one and the same as the insect, that for one with so much talent at winging and soaring and dipping and gliding that life was becoming unreasonably empty and disappointing. The fragile-looking being searched to the length and breadth and height of the world as could be seen through its eyes for something that would make the difference, to perpetuate the enthusiasms of youth. Finally, tired and disillusioned, the dream had the insect creeping back into the darkness of the mythical box, awaiting death.

Then came the dream within the dream, wherein this insect with whom the dreamer identified found itself to be newly-created, with a different kind of skin; with a different, primordial type of energy; and with a special kind of vision, seeing connections more often than separates. Up it flew! (With this new kind of farsighted vision it could be seen that God was not dead, but rather was in need of nurturing.) This form of the insect had a synthesizer in its reproductive system, and after sorting out the most tenable and promising ideas it deposited them with abandon. Many of these then proved themselves fecund as they in their turn rose up into

71

the air to meet with other ideas, infusing each other with newness, begetting new thoughts and new symbols, coming together much as the spectrum of color makes light.

Here it is not appropriate to say "The End," because this may be just the beginning.

SEX IN THE GARDEN
On Identifying Who We Are

There are different ways of approaching questions having to do with vast units of time, especially when we are trying to search out information as to what our heritage has been, as well as to pick up indicators of what our future might be.

Some of us look outward, into the universe. Some of us look downward, into the earth, or even to the very depths of the ocean. Some of us look inward, believing that the mind has its answers even as the heart has its reasons. Remote viewing today gives us previously untold possibilities of perceiving events in other places and other times.

As for me, I choose to look up behind the house, where there is a small piece of land staked out with four twigs and a skinny piece of string—the kitchen garden. If one believes that there is some kind of relationship among all living things, the garden, inhabited by both plant and non-plant life, seems an appropriate place to start the search for meaningful data concerning our heritage. In this small garden we are free to look for clues that will help us put together pieces of the great puzzle of life, for hints suggesting the answers to some of life's great riddles, of whatever nature.

In spite of all the scientific studies that have been done, some of man's most instinctive drives are still unexplained. People talk (and write a lot) about anger, about humor, about religion and politics, but all for the most part remain discussions that are largely rhetorical. The same is true of sex. Today's sex is considered utilitarian for everything from releasing the libido to losing weight. It is also considered to be an art form, in everything from painting to peep-show porn. Sex is "in."

We might get a more meaningful look at sex if we back off from Eighth Avenue and look through a peephole backward through the ages. This particular longitudinal look at sex might be considered caricature, for it started out as a joke. But the comedy writer became the straight woman, and the straight woman became more and more serious with the realization that the considerations involved are no more a joke than life is a joke.

Without evolution, sex could not have proliferated into its many variations of expression. Without sex, evolution's artistry could not have developed with such diversity. Therefore sex and evolution are an appropriate pairing, and it is appropriate that the two topics be considered together. Each aiding and abetting the other, there is a perfect meshing. In this age of unstable relationships, a little of our time might well be put to use in studying this perfect union.

How far have we evolved, sexually speaking? Where are we going, sexually speaking? Just as it is worthwhile in the study of man to look backward in time to the dawn of creation, so might it be well in an analogous fashion to look backward in time to the morning of sex. Starting with the premise that there is a unity among all forms of life, and that man is the most highly-developed species, we begin to realize that by scrutinizing the sexual activity that goes on in forms of life that existed long before we appeared on the scene that in a way we are pinpointing where we have been. Then, by trying to ascertain what is new or different, or indeed, what is the same about our sexual activity, we establish where we are at this particular moment in time in relation to where we have been. Perhaps by using these two points in a projective technique we may be able to ascertain what the future of the sex life of the human being might be, and what implications this might hold for the human being of the future.

As we become students of what goes on in the garden we develop an awareness that there is nothing so bizarre in the behavior of human sexuality that has not been eonian in other forms of life. Our attitudes and activities in the sexual realm may be only echoes of a common prehistoric memory. What are considered by some to be sexual perversions may be no more than archetypal remnants handed down through evolution's kaleidoscope. Some forms of sexual behavior may be archaic residue; others may be harbingers of adjustments to come.

Homo erectus is still so recent in the overall history of life it may be that we have not even begun our most important mutations. With the suggestion being made more frequently by both philosophers and scientists that human beings may be able to choose their own mutations, we had best take a look at the spectrum of possibilities; such a vital part of life as sex is a fitting place to start. By looking backward we may get a better look at the possibilities of the future, recognizing the attributes we want to incorporate or obliterate. The three forms of life which we will study today were populating the earth hundreds of millions of years before man appeared on the scene, and have remained relatively unchanged.

Let us look first at the sexual life of the common garden variety of pea plant, known by its Latin name "pisum sativum." Just as Mendel discovered basic secrets of heredity in his thirty by seven foot garden, cultivating and studying the pea plant, perhaps you and I shall discover secrets of heredity's handmaiden, sex. If we observe the pea plant as it grows and develops, it is like some special kind of adventure. First we see a blossom encircled with tendrils, then we see that the frilly vulva-type flower is complete with clitoris-like equipment; but—look again—this equipment voluptuously enlarges until it becomes a phallic pod! When the pod has matured, erect and proud, it flagrantly bursts open at a touch to release its seed upon the ground, thus starting the cycle over once more, male giving birth to female, female to male, over and over again. One must be awed by the simplicity of the androgynous quality of the pea plant—male and female as one, working together to fulfill one another.

When one dwells on the hypothesis that all forms of life have some kind of interrelationship, as having progressed from some form of common denominator and as continuing to progress on a related continuum, one may begin to consider that perhaps man, who has selectively been strangulating his instinct and feeling for the natural rhythms of life, may find some key in the garden to a birthright of the combination of instinct and intellect. It could be that this attempt to treat as significant what goes on in the garden may be only totemism or anthropomorphism; but there is also the possibility that the utilitarian aspect of the pea plant's cooperative mechanism surviving from cretaceous times could have symbolic implications for us.

But let us get on with our discussion to what some may see as wantonness and perversion. With our next topic you shall be served up not only bizarre behavior but lasciviousness carried to a horrendous extreme. A garden-type spider is our next subject of scrutiny. Mrs. Spider is usually larger than her mate, and she tends to incorporate him—literally. He is put at a disadvantage, but his sexual drive is stronger than the fright growing out of the inborn knowledge of what his fate will be, so lustfully he goes to work.

Masturbating up a bit of semen and placing it on a bit of web, he stuffs the combination into the leg-like appendages on either side of his head. Then, grabbing the female with his other legs he plunges these palpi, sometimes one at a time, sometimes simultaneously in an orgiastic frenzy, into her epigynum or gonopore, her equipment being dependent upon her family connections.

Some spider writers testify that both male and female enjoy these rites of mating; others think that the female just puts up with tradition until it is time for dinner, with the male being the menu. At any rate, they go on through the ages, she playing her macabre role to his furtive and functional role. And so we must ask ourselves—could today's castrating female be the symbolic prototype of Mrs. Spider? Could our modern-day Don Juan be a representation of Mr. Spider and his fear that he must woo, seduce and get away quickly lest seduction be followed by annihilation? Perhaps by seeing some vague similarities between ourselves and these arachnid arthropods we can gain new insights into some of our behaviors.

Moving right along, of all the creatures in the garden the most provocative for any kind of sexual discussion is the snail. Some snails are both sexes at once, some change from one sex to the other, and a few species are strictly female and proliferate through parthenogenesis. If you are a snail, anything goes. The snail that one finds in the garden is probably a close cousin of the Roman snail, the most popular in the annals of expensive restaurants. But before we pluck him up for savoring in a garlicky butter sauce, let's study him, historically speaking. This same snail has left us a great romantic and mythical legacy. Before Cupid was considered responsible for the glint in anyone's eye, this snail was carrying around its own little quiver complete with pointed darts, the better to woo its mate. This archer's equipment is stored in an aperture in the side of the snail's head, the head also housing both penis and vagina.

The stage is set for romance. A large, fleshy foot is raised a bit as the snails meander along their way, and Snail One encounters Snail Two. They meet, touch lips, tentacles and feet, and tenderly caress one another as they sway gently back and forth. As though in response to some kind of evocation, they part and go away one from the other. Then each brings forth a dart from its inlaid quiver and fires it at the other.

The sadist becomes the masochist as the pain inflicted by the darts drives each snail into an erotic frenzy. Speedily, for snails, they rush toward each other. Simultaneously each thrusts its penis into the other's vagina, experiencing mutual orgasm. (Voila, Escargot!) One need not be a great beauty to have the grand passion. But in this evidence that passion is at times ensconced in pain, this residue of sado-masochistic yearning may be perpetuating an archaic misunderstanding of what we like to think of as love. This tale of gastropod love gives us pause.

These three vignettes of what goes on in the garden gives us periscopic vision backward in time. Imagination can give us periscopic vision forward in time. Each phylum and genus and family within both plant and animal worlds has some special characteristic or characteristics setting it apart from others. We humans are no exception.

In acquiring new characteristics, other characteristics are dropped, whatever the species may be. Man, in developing his intellect, has left behind much of what was once instinctive. But that does not mean that the instincts must be lost forever, for the traces are there. Man is the one creature who can transcend himself. He is also conspicuous in nature in that his sex life is not only for reproductive purposes. However, in the weakening of his instincts he is in danger of making sex a cerebral matter. And while man's mind is unique, mind is more than cerebral. One might say that mind is the combining of all man's faculties into an understanding; it is this that supposedly raises him above other forms of life.

As sex becomes more cerebral and mechanical, it may be that the most important part of the human being is left out. Feelings of transcendence are all but eradicated. What could be a celebration of life can become a technique-ridden orgy: object, erections by the hour, orgasms by the score. We cannot transcend ourselves without growing up from our roots, and our deepest taproot, our oldest cultural heritage as human beings, dates back to plant and animal life. We have had time to refine primitive instincts, but trying to eradicate these instincts leaves us poor and passionless. Are we to be machine, or spirit? What are the implications of being human? The way we think and feel about ourselves may well have long-term effects in the sexual realm, as in all others.

It is possible that different mutations of the sexual human being will evolve, depending upon what goes on in individual minds. One mutation, perhaps a behaviorist's dream, might be a creature programmed for maximum efficiency, with built-in skills and a catalogue of information to make the knowledge technologically useful. Another mutation might be a type which bases everything on the chemistry of man, needing only pills to control both inner and outer worlds; and yet another mutation might devote itself simply to sex, looking for pleasure as an end in itself until even that begins to pall.

Sociologists speak of a new mythology growing out of our culture. Will this mythology be based on machines and technology, or one wherein we integrate reason and intuition into a mythology evolving out of untapped human potential?

As much as our children are our progeny, so are our ideas our progeny. Ideas are waiting to be conceived, gestated and born. If we cannot give to sex something that is separately and distinctively human, an intuitive reaching out for an educated instinct, then we are not as clever as the creatures that inhabit our gardens. Perhaps we should go up behind the house, and in that small staked-out piece of land carry on fertility rites dedicated to the birth of new understandings, looking ahead to the best promises that can be hinted at from our own potential and the heritage that we find in the milieu of the kitchen garden.

WORKING WITH NATURE
Chemical vs. Natural Healing

One of the major decisions that we are called on to make as individuals and as a society is whether we will try to control nature or try to cooperate with nature. Let's recognize that there is a world of difference between the necessity for flood control and the depletion of our natural resources for monetary gain, even though it may mean the slow suffocation of the planet. Those responsible for the plundering of the planet have a blind spot. They do not see that we can be only as healthy as our planet is healthy. Just one of the issues of control or cooperation has to do not only with our bodies, but with our psyches.

Today in psychiatry the aim of mending mental aberration is to control the psyche by alleviating symptoms with psychomarmacological agents. There is a pill for depression, a pill for anxiety. But an important concept is being neglected, which is that given the opportunity, we may have vast resources ourselves, to mend ourselves. By cooperating with nature rather than trying to control it we could be freed from what at times has come to be the tyranny of the psychiatric community. We have adopted neglect of our intuition for the sedation delivered by the drug companies. Individuals can be made psychologically ill by a lack of integrity in the dictates of an unwell environment. While moral support would be a more natural means of improving a psychological prognosis, it has instead become habit to prescribe medication to control all those unpopular feelings.

The reason that pharmacology has taken such a strong hold is that it has been possible to identify that there is such a thing as a chemical disorder of the brain. But what is not being recognized is that trauma alters the chemistry of the brain and that this can be countered by "undoing" the effects of the trauma. There is evidence that psychotherapy can provide chemical changes, undoing the chemical imbalance, by getting at the cause of the disease rather than just treating the symptoms. In other words, helping patients to feel understood can be a more useful tool than pills. And the dream can help us get to new understandings.

At times, with the help of dreams, we can solve some of our problems that have seemed insurmountable by giving us access to the reservoir of the Unconscious. Eli Whitney, inventor of the cotton gin, and Elias Howe, inventor of the sewing machine, represent just two examples of dreams being the inspiration for a solution that would make the invention functional. Friedrich Kakule, as a result of the help he received from his dreams, figured out how the benzine ring was formed. Niels Bohr is reported to have won the Nobel Prize in Physics in 1922 as the result of an enlightening dream; Otto Loewi won the Nobel Prize in Medicine in 1936 for the discovery of the secret of nerve impulses, revealed to him in two different dreams.

These are just a few examples of the power of dreams. Everyday insights inspired by dreams can be just as important. Emanuel Donchin of the University of Illinois has done research positing that 99% of motivation comes from the Unconscious. This is a reminder that much of the time our conscious mind does not know why it is doing what it is doing. The dream, if we can learn its language, can help us understand what we are all about. The dream is a natural aid to our mental health, whereas medication is often like bludgeoning our sensibilities to ape a sense of normalcy. One of the most important axioms we are in danger of losing in our technological society is that we do have mending capacities of our own. We need to have more faith in ourselves and in our transcendent abilities. The ingestion of man-made chemicals, rather than just being a quick fix, is dulling our self-healing sensitivities.

THE DREAM AS QUARK
Alternative Realities

"Quark" is a word coined by James Joyce in *Finnegan 's Wake:* "Three quarks for Muster Mark." The word "quark" was later adopted by physicists at the suggestion of a fellow physicist as an appropriate word for theories concerning subatomic particles. Quark was a word that was needed; quarks came to represent the equivalent of smaller units in the atom.

Why might "quarks" be important to us? Harald Fritsch in his book *Quarks* pointed out that the laws of quantum theory set an absolute limit on our ability to predict. Using this as a guide, it explains why time and time gain, when evidence points to someone having only six months to live, that they prove to be the exception to the medical prognosis, and they can be found to be hale and hearty many years later. And why people who have been told they will be mentally ill for the rest of their lives can prove that they have grown to be stable and competent. It is the window of uncertainty exemplified by the quark that gives us the possibility of a window of change.

The dream has much in common with the quark, and might even be considered to be a version of a quark. The dream can help us to know things that we do not know in waking hours. The dream can tell us something about the nature of the spirit. It is not a big jump to believe that a wounded spirit is the precursor not only of physical illness, but of emotional illness as well. Positive or negative changes in spirit can change physical and emotional health. Once we are helped to new understandings, positive changes can begin to happen.

Because we all have problems seeing as real things that we cannot see or hear or smell or touch, the quark, along with the dream, appears to be something which is unimportant except for philosophical discussion. But as the quark is representative of three building blocks of the atom, it is also representative of the relationship of body, spirit and mind to matter. If we are more machine than spirit, we are susceptible only to the uncertainties of the vagaries of quantum theory. If we are more spirit than machine, we can be influential to some degree in affecting our surroundings. We can alter our environment, using spirit to promote a negative entropy, promoting harmony, and even changing matter. Remarkable tales of prayer affecting nature are heard from time to time. Feats of superhuman strength are occasionally reported. It seems that miracles do exist. When Jesus cured a blind man, giving him back his sight, he is reported to have said, "These things that I do, so can ye do, and more."

Our physical health benefits when modern medicine tunes in to the concept of the spirit needing attention, as well as the physical body. This is true of emotional illness as well, which is supposedly the result of "a broken brain." Stress tends to be the biggest single factor in causing illness, yet the significance of the importance of spirit is bypassed in both etiology and prognosis. "Keeping our spirits up" is more than a saying.

Sometimes the best therapy can be done with a look, and great harm can be done with a look. The subtleties of personal relationships are powerful. We send off positive or negative energy without being aware of it. We are sometimes barraged by a sense of turbulence around some people, and enveloped in a sense of calm by others. Talk therapy does not cure by words alone.

Keeping quarks in mind can help us to bend reality to our specifications. Words, looks, dreams, can be steered toward bringing about positive changes, using ideas embodied in the common, or uncommon, quark.

MULTIPLE
PERSONALITY DISORDER
Family Therapy

Also called Dissociative Identity Disorder, there has been much more written about the characteristics of Multiple Personality Disorder or Dissociative Identity Disorder than has been written about the cure. Most of the formulas for treatment have been to get the personalities in touch with each other through hypnosis in order to achieve eventual integration. Just as the personalities split off as the result of trauma, making the "Center" aware of other personalities is like introducing members of a family to one another, until finally the family is the person.

We all have different states of mind. We may be a happy person one day, one moment, and a sad person another day, another moment—the same for angry, whimsical, and whatever. With the multiply traumatized those states can become individuals, complete with their own particular idiosyncratic illnesses, eye prescriptions, handwriting, walking gaits, etc. Just the fact that different personalities have different illnesses and even different eye colors is testament to the ability of the individual to change.

While hypnosis has been the main tool in working with dissociative personalities, there may be another paradigm within which to work to bring about a healing, a knitting together of the seams of a broken personality. What seems more apparent now than previously is that at least with some of the splintered personalities, the selves can be seen as personifications of feelings. It is not just a case of a new personality being forged when an experience is traumatically burned into the brain, but that the feelings which have been inspired by untenable situations are solidified into personalities which express those feelings. Altogether the different selves make an interesting family. Some members of this family are not kindly thought of by other members of the family. While it does seem important to find the "Center," that may not be as important as working with each member of this invented family of personalities.

If consistent trauma involving all kinds of abuse would shatter a person, might there not be ways to work with a different set of relationships and a different environment? Reintegration of the individual might have a corollary in the idea of a dysfunctional family learning to integrate. Learning to trust must come first, and this will be difficult, but not impossible. Working with each of the shattered personalities separately, individually, could be the equivalent of discovering that although disparate ideas are represented, the ideas are representative of one mind. As each of the personalities begins to feel understood, it opens the possibility of cooperation between and among the personalities. As dissociations begin to meld together the concept "All is One" becomes a unifying tool.

And healing can be a combination of different factors: One, the paradigm suggested by Norman Cousins' dramatic recovery from a type of muscular disease which was considered fatal: If stress makes one ill, he reasoned, why wouldn't the opposite of stress be curative? Megavitamin therapy, humor and relaxation, along with an indomitable spirit, brought him to an ultimate recovery and new career as a medical consultant.

An amalgam of healing techniques may prove to be appropriate in working with any particular illness, including Dissociative Disorders. Although only peripherally dealing with Dissociative Disorders, Dr. Fredric Schiffer's work with Dual Brain Psychology has established that significantly often, one hemisphere is "the mature mind," and the opposite hemisphere is "the immature mind." Because of the information elicited in split brain studies Dr. Schiffer was able to establish the existence of two separate selves represented by the two separate hemispheres, thus enabling him to work with the mature self toward a healthier personality. This may well prove to be an important tool in helping multiple personalities to integrate. Knowing which is the "stronger" of the neocortical hemispheres could be a powerful ally.

Just as a whole family begins to change if one person in a family changes, so could it be with the family that is organized within one person. Also, even though it may be well hidden, within every person is a wish to get well. Multimodal therapy can access different aspects of the traumatic foundation on which the illness has built itself. Art therapy, play therapy, music therapy, aroma therapy, good food, exercise, rest, all play a part in reconstituting a healthy multi-modal self. Multiple personalities use artistic expression as avenues of self integration. The demands made on their self-healing abilities often help to finely hone natural artistic and intellectual gifts.

Because so much of trauma is held in the body, body work should not be neglected. A sixty-five year old man in New York City who had been in therapy for years had not changed, overly concerned with keeping everything "in check." On the advice of a friend he tried massage therapy, and in his first session he began to sob convulsively. From there on he began to know his feelings, and from there on he rebuilt his life. The effects of physical abuse which he had not been able to consciously remember had been held captive in his body, and were able to be released by the massage therapist's touch.

With multiple personalities there has usually been horrendous physical abuse, along with psychological abuse. Physical and emotional scars are often somatized, so that body therapy can be extremely helpful. A Reiki therapist is able to access old hurts, sometimes even without touch. A young woman who had been treated by a Reiki Master began to self heal, and began to be able to organize her many selves, in time becoming a Reiki Master herself. The creative instinct which had been used to deal with trauma by inventing separate personalities had been able to apply itself to a reworking, to integration.

From talk therapy to play therapy to art therapy to massage or Reiki, body and spirit can help those with multiple personalities to detoxify.

ON ATTITUDE
An Identity Crisis

One of the problems that has come out of the complications of the way the brain is organized is that we have learned to identify with our inventions, fostering the tendency to worship technology. It would be more appropriate to pay homage to that part of ourselves that invents and creates rather than to honor the invention. The irony is great. Rather than focusing attention on the human being's capabilities for bringing about changes, it is as though we have no choice. Our inventions get out of hand, the individual tends to feel helpless, and we become the pawns of our own creations.

It appears that we have a problem <u>realizing</u> ourselves as well as we realize our creations.   Who are we? Is the individual an animal, a machine, a god, or what? We cannot act appropriately without knowing what sort of creature we are. Interpreting our animal nature as base, finding competition with machines unfulfilling, and discovering that trying to act like a god is impossible as well as presumptuous, it may be that being a human being involves a high tolerance for ambiguity and a great deal of patience. The attitude with which we approach the philosophical equation of the relationship of ourselves to life can make the difference between self-destruction and the possibility of gaining the whole world in a way that so far has only been hinted at.

With the beginning of a new awareness of an inner self the individual is approaching the exploration of what Theodore Reik called "the last dark continent." Over the span of years, from Descartes' "I think, therefore I am," to the study of ways to explore the new frontier, that previously undefined self is beginning to gain an identity. It is with such an attitude that the new world starts to open up, that our knowledge grows, and that our insights and understandings begin to reach levels previously only dimly suspected as being within the realm of possibility. Because of what has been called "the heyday of science" we have had an attitude of not believing in anything that could not be seen or measured. Now, reaching for new definitions, we discover a generator within ourselves; with this generator we are going to have to "feel" our way to a new set of attitudes to be in keeping with the new definitions. We have been all wrapped up in the idea of Mind. The new definition has something to do not only with Mind, and with Body, but with Spirit. An awareness of attitude cannot be overemphasized. We are beginning to recognize that our Unconscious may be our best friend.

When one is in the market for a new car, cars begin to be noticed more than before. When one is interested in buying a house, houses are noticed as never before. Attitude determines just where attention is focused. Now, as we are beginning to shift our psychic attention to a combination of internal and external matters, we are on the brink of a major new development in the growth of the human being. What was once the province of the poet is becoming fair game for the man in the street. Choose your attitude, you choose a set of understandings, and you choose your direction for growth.

A wise friend remarked, "It's where you're going that's important, not how fast you're getting there." Generally, we don't seem to like where we're going, and yet we are rushing to get there. There is a defense mechanism called "Identification with the Aggressor," which sometimes gets in our way. As though it gives us power, we sometimes try to be like those who are in power. This defense explains why, for instance, children will tend to take on the violent actions of a violent parent—if they are like the offending parent, there is an unconscious belief that the same behavior will be a protection from being a victim of violent behavior oneself. Unfortunately, it is sometimes easier to adopt the value system of those in power than to live by a different value system.

We have been in denial about what is happening to Earth, to Gaia. And because our world of technology is murdering our environment, we had better make sure that we do not identify with the people in power who have little or no regard for Nature, and that the people we choose to be in charge of our planet have respect for all living things, especially Earth.

Consciousness is what we pay attention to. The more that we become conscious that we have a complementary thought system—an alternative possibility—the more our focus will shift in our perception of day-to-day living, especially important in our problem-solving technique. Attitude runs in tandem with consciousness and can be all important in helping us to expand our consciousness to draw more on the attitudes of the thinking style of the right hemisphere.

We do not have to take anything away from the marvelous array of talents of the left brain—except for the leadership role. The more we learn about the characteristics of each of the thinking styles available to us, it becomes clear that we need to find ways to put the part of us in charge that is the expert in seeing the whole picture. The more that we become aware of the possibilities available to us, the more we will be able to take the risk of making our left-brain characteristics subordinate to our right brain "higher power."

Just being aware of the gifts of the silent hemisphere will be the strongest aid in helping us depend more on this hemisphere. And there are specific things we can do to encourage this dependence. For example, before ready to go to sleep at night, write on a piece of paper what question you would like answered. When waking in the morning, search your mind for dream residue. Also, take time to meditate or to daydream. Run, rather than jog. Sing, play music. If you are quite certain that your brain is classically organized (left hemisphere, reductionist; right hemisphere, holistic) try breathing while covering the right nostril, thus giving more oxygen power to the relatively silent right hemisphere. Make of it what you will: In one dream seminar a woman reported that she had "fortune cookie" dreams whenever she slept on her left side.

SPERRY
Science and Moral Priority

Roger Sperry's book *Science and Moral Priority* escaped my attention until after most of the essays in *Wrong Way Brain* had been completed. As I read Sperry's book it was like a personal endorsement, for in his book he lays the groundwork for the importance of recognizing the qualities that brain researchers in the years after Sperry were able to define and redefine—that is, the values that Sperry talked about as being the province of what in most people is the right hemisphere. Sperry says in simple sentences what I was trying to convey, one way or another, in each of my essays.

Without Sperry's work on the split-brain experiments most of my essays would not have been written. Although Sperry and his followers were able to identify the different thinking qualities of the two hemispheres, *Science and Moral Priority* is mainly about the importance of recognizing a value system, although it does not specifically identify the value system as being the province of the right hemisphere. Sperry does acknowledge that value judgments lie outside the realm of science, which he acknowledges does not always see the whole picture. Sperry recognized the different thinking styles of the two hemispheres, yet there had not yet been time for the significance of the differences to be appreciated.

Although Sperry led the way to the configurations of right/left hemisphere differences with his split brain studies, he does not address this in *Science and Moral Priority*. What he does do is to recognize the importance of what later turned out to be right brain interests, especially values. He makes a strong case for the need of science to incorporate a sense of values into its rubric. He also discusses the importance of individual thought—independent thinking—acknowledging that science tends to be "closed in." Recognizing that what a person or a society values determines what he, she or it does, he talks about the perception of "the whole picture" seen by left brain interests turning out to be a contradiction in terms, as the concept of the whole picture is one of the interests of the right hemisphere.

Sperry sees science as being reductionist. Often the values of society are not based on a whole-picture view but on narrow views of self interest. Also, he gives further importance to the thinking of the right hemisphere without specifically giving the right hemisphere credit by saying, "Our subjective values...not only <u>reflect</u> environmental conditions but also <u>produce and control</u> them." In other words, we create our environment. Which is why the holistic thinking of right hemisphere is of such vital importance.

Scientists rely heavily on left-brain skills. As much as Sperry was thinking in terms of science as being the strongest suit to save us and our planet, he recognizes that there may be something missing that needs amending. It was of great comfort to the author of *Wrong Way Brain* that, even though we do not use exactly the same words, the same topics are discussed. Reading *Science and Moral Priority* was like getting a pat on the back from the individual who was the most significant mentor in giving the gift of the building blocks of a somewhat passionate philosophical stance.

Sperry speaks of the integrity of nature. He talks about a lot of things as being important that are things that have since the writing of his book (early eighties) turned out to be recognized as attributes of the right hemisphere. He has a telling, though succinct, sub-chapter on "The Neglected Minor Hemisphere." And he recognizes that a quick grasp of the whole may be found preferable to a logical sequential approach—(a right hemisphere specialty being preferable to what tends to be the logical sequential approach of the left hemisphere.) And he supports a revised philosophy in which modern (non-reductive) science becomes the most effective and reliable means available for determining valid criteria for moral value and meaning. In other words, he is saying that science needs to be guided by tenets which more and more have been proved by researchers who came after Sperry to be the province of the right hemisphere.

Time and research have been able to clarify the differences in the way the two hemispheres think. Viewpoints advocated in the essays in *Wrong Way Brain* are largely the result of work that was done by Sperry's colleagues following Sperry's work and following the publication of his book. The seeds for the thinking that came after Sperry's seminal work are in his book. The focus of thinking is the same. Sperry beautifully distills what has become clear to those who follow him. He wrote, "What is needed...is a new ethic... that will make it sacrilegious to deplete natural resources, to pollute the environment, to overpopulate, to erase or degrade other species, or to otherwise destroy, demean, or defile the evolving quality of the biosphere, etc." Perhaps the "etc." will be recognized as being the foundation of the essays in *Wrong Way Brain*.

THE END

Selected Bibliography

Andreasen, Nancy C., M.D. *The Broken Brain*. New York: Harper & Row, 1984.

Avorn, Jerry, M.D. *Powerful Medicines. The Benefits, Risks and Cost of Prescription Drugs*. New York: Knopf, 2004

Bateson, Gregory. *Mind and Nature: A Necessary Unity*. New York: Bantam Books, 1979.

Bergland, Richard, M.D. *The Fabric of Mind*. New York: Viking Penguin Inc., 1985.

Bergson, Henri. *Creative Evolution*. New York: Random House, 1944 (originally published 1911.)

Blakeslee, Thomas R. *The Attitude Factor: Extend Your Life by Changing the Way You Think*. London: Thorsons/Harper Collins, 1997.

Blakeslee, Thomas R. *Beyond the Conscious Mind: Unlocking the Secrets of the Self*. New York: Plenum Press, 1996.

Blakeslee, Thomas R. *The Right Brain*. Garden City, NY: Anchor Press, 1980.

Bogen, Joseph E., M.D. and Bogen, Glenda M. "The Other Side of the Brain III: The Corpus Callosum and Creativity." *Bulletin of the Los Angeles Neurological Societies*. October 1969, Vol. 34, No. 4.

Breggin, Peter, M.D., "Psychopharmacology and Human Values." *Journal of Humanistic Psychology*. Spring 2003, Vol. 43, No. 2.

Breggin, Peter, M.D. and Cohen, David. *Your Drug May Be Your Problem*. Reading, MA: Perseus Books, 1999.

Cameron, Norman. *Personality Development and Psychopathology*, Boston, MA: Houghton Mifflin Company, 1963.

Capra, Fritjof. *The Tao of Physics*. New York: Bantam Books, 1976.

Carr, Donald. *The Forgotten Senses*. Garden City, NY: Doubleday, 1972.

Carson, Rachel. *The Sense of Wonder*. New York: Harper & Row, 1965.

Cutter, Rebecca. *When Opposites Attract*. New York: Penguin Books, 1994.

Diamond, Stephen A. *Anger, Madness and the Daimonic*. Albany: State University of New York Press, 1996.

Drimmer, Frederick, ed. *The Animal Kingdom*. Vol. III. Garden City, NY: Doubleday& Co., 1954.

Diagnostic and Statistical Manual of Mental Disorders (DSM-IV.) Fourth Edition. Washington, *DC:* American Psychiatric Association, 1994.

Edwards, Betty. *Drawing on the Right Side of the Brain*. Los Angeles, CA: J. P. Tarcher, Inc., 1979.

Ferguson, Marilyn. *The Aquarian Conspiracy*. Los Angeles, CA: J. P. Tarcher, Inc., 1980.

Fox, Matthew and Sheldrake, Rupert. *Natural Grace. Dialogues on Creation, Darkness, and the Soul in Spirituality and Science*. New York: Doubleday, 1996.

Fromm, Erich. *The Revolution of Hope Toward a Humanized Technology*. New York: Harper & Row, 1968.

Freud, Sigmund. *Three Essays on the Theory of Sexuality*. New York: Avon Books, 1962.

Gerber, Richard, M.D. *Vibrational Medicine*. 3rd edition. Rochester, Vermont: Bear & Co., 2001.

Guralnik, David B., editor. *Webster's New World Dictionary*. 2nd College Edition. United States: World Publishing Company, 1978.

Gustaitis, Rasa. *Turning On*. New York: The Macmillan Co., 1969.

Hirstein, William. *Brain Fiction: Self-Deception and the Riddle of Confabulation*. Cambridge, MA: Massachusetts Institute of Technology, 2005.

Hormiga, Gustavo. *Higher Level Phylogenetics of Erigonine Spiders (Araneae, Linyphiidae, Erigoninae.)* Washington, D.C.: Smithsonian Institution Press, 2000.

Hunt, Morton. *The Universe Within*. New York: Simon and Schuster, 1982.

Hyman, Stanley E. *Darwin for Today*. New York: Viking Press, 1963.

Jantsch, Erich. *The Self-Organizing Universe*. Elmsford, NY: Pergamon Press, 1980.

Joseph, R. *The Right Brain and the Unconscious*. New York: Plenum Press, 1992.

Jung, C. G. *Memories, Dreams, Reflections*. New York: Random House, 1965.

Koestler, Arthur. *The Ghost in the Machine*. New York: Random House, 1976.

Kramer, Peter. *Listening to Prozac*. New York: Viking, 1993.

Kuhn, Thomas S. *The Structure of Scientific Revolutions*. Second Edition. Chicago: University of Chicago Press, 1970.

Kutchins, Herb and Kirk, Stuart A. *Making Us Crazy. DSM: The Psychiatric Bible and the Creation of Mental Disorders*. New York: The Free Press, Simon & Schuster Inc., 1997.

Langer, Susanne K. *Philosophy in a New Key*. Cambridge, MA: Harvard University Press, 1967.

Lovelock, James. *Gaia, A New Look at Life on Earth*. Guernsey, G.B.: Oxford University Press, 1979.

Lovelock, James. *The Ages of Gaia, A Biography of Our Living Earth*. New York: W.W. Norton & Co., 1988.

Luhrman, T. M. *Of Two Minds, The Growing Disorder in American Psychiatry*. New York: Alfred A. Knopf, 2000.

Maslow, Abraham. *Toward a Psychology of Being*. Second Edition. Princeton, NJ: D. VanNostrand Company, Inc., 1968.

May, Rollo. *The Courage to Create*. New York: W. W. Norton, 1975.

McGreal, Ian P., editor. *Great Thinkers of the Western World*. New York: Harper Collins, 1992.

Newbold, Heather, Ed. *Life Stories. World-Renowned Scientists Reflect on Their Lives and the Future of Life on Earth*. Berkeley, CA: University of California Press, 2000.

Ornstein, Robert E., editor. *The Nature of Human Consciousness*. San Francisco: W. H. Freeman and Company, 1973.

Ornstein, Robert. *The Right Mind: Making Sense of the Hemispheres*. New York: Harcourt Brace & Company, 1979.

Pekkanen, John. *The American Connection*. Chicago, IL: Follett Publishing Co., 1973.

Pert, Candace. *The Molecules of Emotion. The Science behind Mind-Body Medicine*. New York: Simon & Schuster, 1999.

Petersen, Kai. *Prehistoric Life on Earth*. New York: E. P. Dutton & Co., Inc., 1961.

Restak, Richard M., M.D. *The Brain, The Last Frontier*. New York: Warner Books, 1979.

Samples, Bob. *The Mind of Our Mother*. Boulder, CO: Addison-Wesley, 1981.

Schiffer, Fredric, M.D. *Of Two Minds, The Revolutionary Science of Dual-Brain Psychology*. New York. The Free Press, 1998.

Servan-Schreiber, David, M.D. *The Instinct to Heal. Curing Stress, Anxiety and Depression without Drugs and without Talk Therapy*. Paris, France: Editions Robert Laffont, 2003. Distributed by St. Martin's Press.

Sheldrake, Rupert. *Seven Experiments That Could Change the World*. New York: Riverhead Books, 1995.

Shlain, Leonard. *The Alphabet Versus the Goddess*. New York: Penguin Putnam Inc., 1998.

Sire, Marcel. *Secrets of Plant Life*. New York: Viking Press, 1969.

Sperry, Roger, M.D. "Lateral Specialization of Cerebral Function in the Surgically Separated Hemispheres." *The Psychophysiology of Thinking*. Edited by F. J. McGuigan and R. A. Schoonover. New York: Academic Press, 1973.

Sperry, Roger, M.D. *Science and Moral Priority*. New York: Columbia University Press, 1983.

Ullman, Montague, M.D., and Zimmerman, Nan. *Working with Dreams*. New York: Dell Publishing Co., 1979.

Vaughan, Susan C, M.D. *The Talking Cure: The Science Behind Psychotherapy*. New York; Grossett/Putnam, 1997.

Vitale, Barbara Meister. *Free Flight, Celebrating Your Right Brain*. Rolling Hills Estates, C A: Jalmar Press, 1986.

Whitman, Walt. *Leaves of Grass*. New York: Rinehart & Co., 1949.

Wonder, Jacquelyn and Donovan, Priscilla. *Whole Brain Thinking*, New York: William Morrow and Company, 1984.

Zinn, Howard. *The Twentieth Century, A People's History*. New York: Harper Perennial, 1998.